Merry Christmas, 2000!

Enjoy the Book, G-I Doc

Your friend,
Geri Doc

PEREZ ON MEDICINE

THE WHIMSICAL ART OF
JOSE S. PEREZ

TEXT BY
WAYMAN R. SPENCE, M.D.

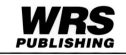

WRS
PUBLISHING

A Division of WRS Group, Inc.
Waco, Texas

First published in the United States of America in 1993
by WRS Publishing, A Division of WRS Group, Inc.,
701 N. New Road, Waco, Texas 76710.
Book design by Kenneth Turbeville.
Jacket design by Joe James.

Printed in Hong Kong

10 9 8 7 6 5 4 3 2

Library of Congress Cataloging-in-Publication Data

Perez, Jose S., 1929-
    Perez on medicine / art of Jose S. Perez ; text by Wayman R. Spence.
        p.   cm.
    ISBN 1-56796-005-7 : $29.95
    1. Perez, Jose S., 1929-   . 2. Medicine in art. 3. Medicine—Specialists and
specialties—Caricatures and cartoons.
    I. Spence, Wayman R., 1934-   . II. Title.
    ND237.P362A4 1993
    759.13—dc20
                                                    93-10421
                                                      CIP

This book is dedicated to all members of the medical
profession who have helped many sufferers not only to
endure, but often to be healed.

I intend my art to be an expressive way to penetrate to
the truth. Invariably, there is more than one side to a
story, especially when science and art are practiced in a
free society. Satirical artists have always used their art to
identify and help reform frailties, something for which I
hope sufferers and healers alike are grateful. We all need
to laugh at what we fear, and nothing today is more
troubling than disability and death.

Jose Perez

TABLE OF CONTENTS

FOREWORD

The paintings in this collection came into being somewhat by serendipity. As an art collector and medical historian, I discovered Perez' work through a professional contact and, partly because I have two sons who are lawyers, purchased a painting from him which irreverently satirized a day in court. Several months later, I asked Perez if he could do a painting for me satirically analyzing psychiatry. I had almost specialized in psychiatry after medical school and always enjoyed the subject. When I received his painting of the psychiatrist, I decided to have him do another painting about a part of medicine with which I had had recent personal experience as a suffering patient. He painted "The Emergency Room," and by then I was hooked on his genius and couldn't stop. One painting led to another over the next three years as Perez and I undertook in earnest an analysis of all the branches of modern-day medicine.

Upon viewing the paintings and drawings of Jose Perez shown in this book, students of art and medical history invariably compare his work with the great artists of the past whose good-natured humor, and sometimes savage ridicule, satirized pre–twentieth century medicine. Boilly, Cruikshank, Daumier, Gillray, Hogarth, Kley, and Rowlandson all can be seen in the style and feel of Perez' work. But Perez has enjoyed a distinct advantage over these earlier artists, because, by virtue of his time in history, he has had a relative freedom from earlier religious dogmas and superstitions. He has also been able to separate the world of medicine into its many modern-day specialties, each with its own personality and perspectives.

Jose Perez has seized the opportunity to take up the torch from the greatest satirical artists of the past at a time when relationships between sufferers and their healers are undergoing unprecedented changes.

Many infamous diseases from the past have all but disappeared, and others are on the run, exiting stage left. Lifestyle is the magic ingredient in the etiology of today's most notable diseases. Heart attacks, cancer, and AIDS are blamed on the way we live, not on the gods or even microbes. The patient is now recognized by both sufferers and healers to be perhaps the most important member of the health-care team. Medical ethics is debated on our front pages, and death with dignity is a sought-after right.

The drawings preceding each of Perez' paintings show some of the experimentation and developmental thought he went through with each subject. Sometimes the simple sketches are as much fun to view as his detailed paintings, which are intricate oils on canvas that communicate different messages to different people at different times. In one frame of mind, one can view his art with gentle humor, and at another time, be moved to reform a frailty or outright deception.

At first glance, it may appear that some of Perez' art treats too disrespectfully those who do so much to preserve life and health. But his satire is intended to prod the viewer to question and think about many of the more serious issues confronting our health-care system today. His art is a mirror irreverently reflecting our reality. He often paints physicians as male, nurses as subservient, and patients as stooges, not because he wants it that way, but because that is the way it has been.

Enjoy **Perez on Medicine** for its obvious tongue-in-cheek humor, but let Perez' art, my written interpretations, and your own experiences with life and death lead you to meaningful insights into the countless useful metaphors of his socially relevant work.

Wayman R. Spence, M.D.

INTRODUCING JOSE PEREZ

With a personality as unique as his art, Jose Perez has painted his way through life. His paintings are his voice, his method of expressing himself, his commentary on society.

Born in Houston, Texas, on June 30, 1929, of Mexican parents, Perez moved with his family to Mexico when he was five years old. Returning to the United States as a teenager, Perez swam across the border carrying the papers which proved he was a U.S. citizen. His brother, also a U.S. citizen, had lost his papers and so talked Jose into swimming back to their country. This incident is a foreshadowing of the personality Perez was to become.

Jose developed a sense of humor in his early years, and it's been an integral part of his life and his art ever since. Through years of working in menial jobs, through his struggle for recognition as an artist, through a bout with glaucoma—through all the trying times of his life, Jose Perez has maintained his sense of humor.

His career has evolved rather than developed. While Perez was working as a busboy, Mrs. Ruth Ford Van Dyke, owner and director of the Chicago Academy, noticed the drawings he had done on the backs of discarded menus. Mrs. Van Dyke invited Perez to study art at the academy and, within a few months, under the guidance of Louis Grell, a noted muralist, Perez was given a scholarship. He also studied with Allen St. John and William Mosby at the American Academy in Chicago.

Various events have interrupted his pursuit of art as a profession. In 1951,

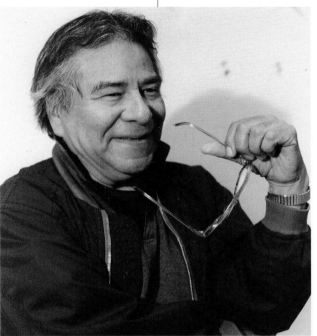

Perez was drafted into the army. After serving two years, he returned to the American Academy and studied art for another two years. He spent the next few years drifting from place to place, working at odd jobs—as a strawberry picker in Oregon, a construction worker in Houston, and a factory handyman in Chicago.

Then, in 1958, he wandered to Washington, D.C., where he found the art ambience stimulating and where he started to paint professionally. His first art commission was to paint a series of large paintings depicting the American Revolution for the Drummer Boy Museum in Cape Cod, Massachusetts.

The confusion Perez had felt in earlier years evaporated when he began to concentrate on satirical art and pursue his profession seriously. His work is owned by a wide variety of art collectors in the United States and Europe, and in 1981, Houston, Texas declared a Jose S. Perez Day for its distinguished native artist.

Perez says of his own work: "Satirical painting suits my need as an artist: The freedom to distort and yet remain in the spectrum of the fine arts. It is also my best way to communicate with my fellow man. The social comment, in which satirical art expresses its power, is without malice; it merely represents my personal view of the world as I see it, either from an historical point, the present, or the future."

This is just a brief glimpse of Jose Perez. For a real introduction, take a close look at his art—the eyes, the heart, and the soul of Jose Perez.

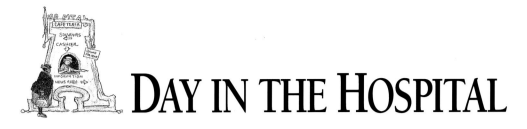

A DAY IN THE HOSPITAL

This masterfully complex painting sets the stage for Perez' series on medicine. It is not just a story about doctors, because Perez does not treat medicine as the exclusive turf of doctors. Rather, it shows the inescapable relationships between healers, sufferers, disease, and death. The conglomerate that brings these components together is what we call our health-care system. In reality, it should be called our illness-care system. This painting holds up a mirror to the very essence of the system—our hospitals.

After focusing on the large, central doctor, one's eye is tempted to move in all directions to scenes and sub-scenes throughout the canvas. But, if you will, first look at the doctor's facial expression and body language. This very human figure seems to be wondering what in the world he should do with all the suffering humanity he confronts.

The patient on the operating table—who looks as if he's just about to expire—is getting a lot of attention from the medical staff. Merlin the Magician is positioned next to the patient, perhaps to help him cross the River Styx. Is all this care too late? Would it be wiser to free up the doctors to help patients with better chances of survival?

The priest-like fellow in the purple robe holds a burning candle, perhaps trying to shed light on the situation, or maybe suggesting that modern medicine is closer to that of past centuries than we like to think. One hundred years from now, will blood transfusions, scalpels, and radiation-scattering X-rays seem as primitive as bleeding and purging seem to us? Will the depersonalized treatment of patients—shown by the robot being oiled—result in robot-like people, who take no responsibility for their own care?

Animal rights activists will identify with the orangutan holding the placard, while the children below him remind us that children have rights, too, and not to be abused is one of those rights.

As the Grim Reaper in the lower right-hand corner comes to claim his prey, we realize that the wisdom of Solomon could not solve the needs of modern society with all its pressure groups, here shown by the demonstrators in the hall balcony. Perez himself is seen painting on a crumbling wall the words, "Les Misérables," an apt description of the patients in our system, and something of a double entendre: Perez' daughter spent two years traveling with the Broadway musical of that name.

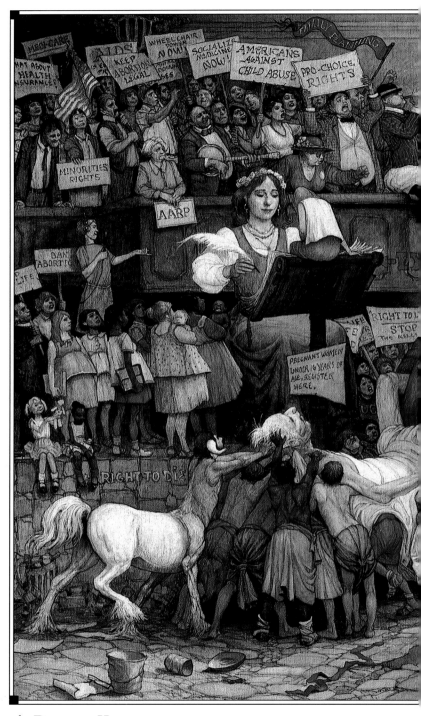

A Day in the Hospital – 48" x 96" (123cm x 246cm)

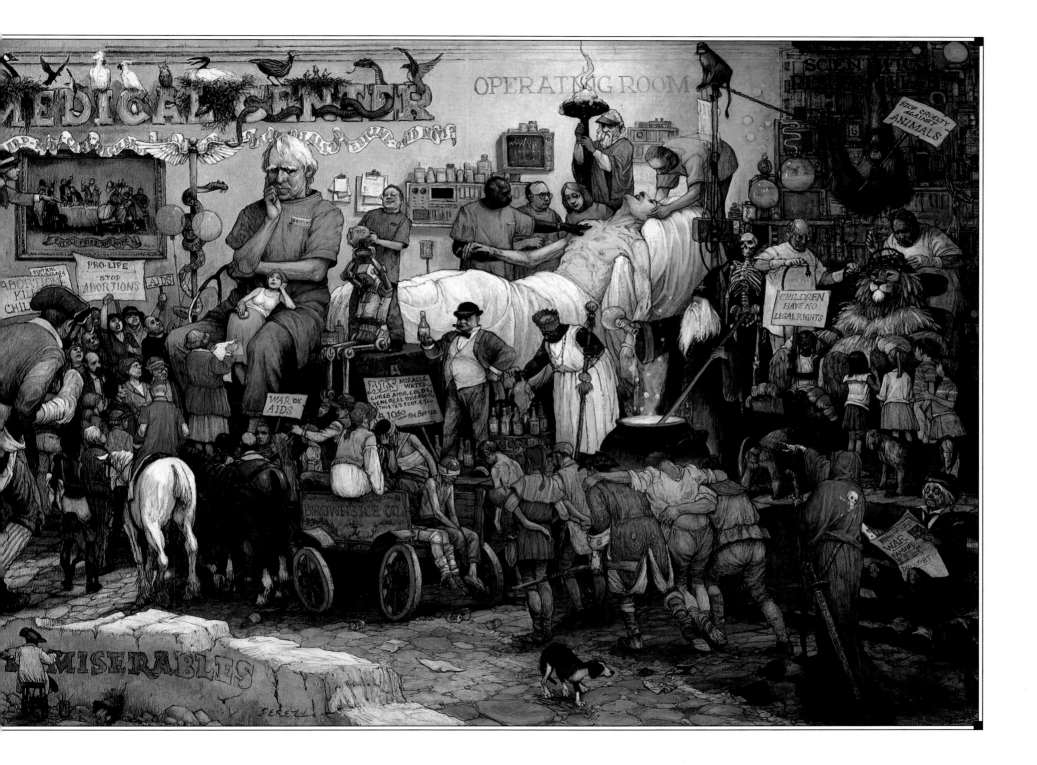

THE 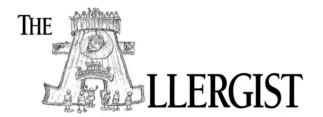LLERGIST

In this painting, Perez chose not to include a doctor— perhaps because a patient with allergies often endures the battle alone. Anyone with allergies can appreciate the plight of the patient. The poor, red-nosed man cowers in his bed, helplessly spraying bug repellent while the army of invading warriors— pollution, pollen, and dust mites—relentlessly marches on him.

These miniature tormentors seem likely to win the battle, causing their prey's mucous membranes to swell and itch. And when the warriors have finished their work, they will probably retreat and camp somewhere nearby, perhaps under the pillows or bed sheets, to rest before attacking again.

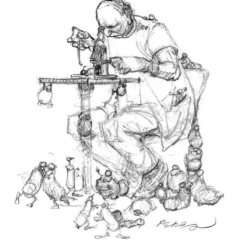

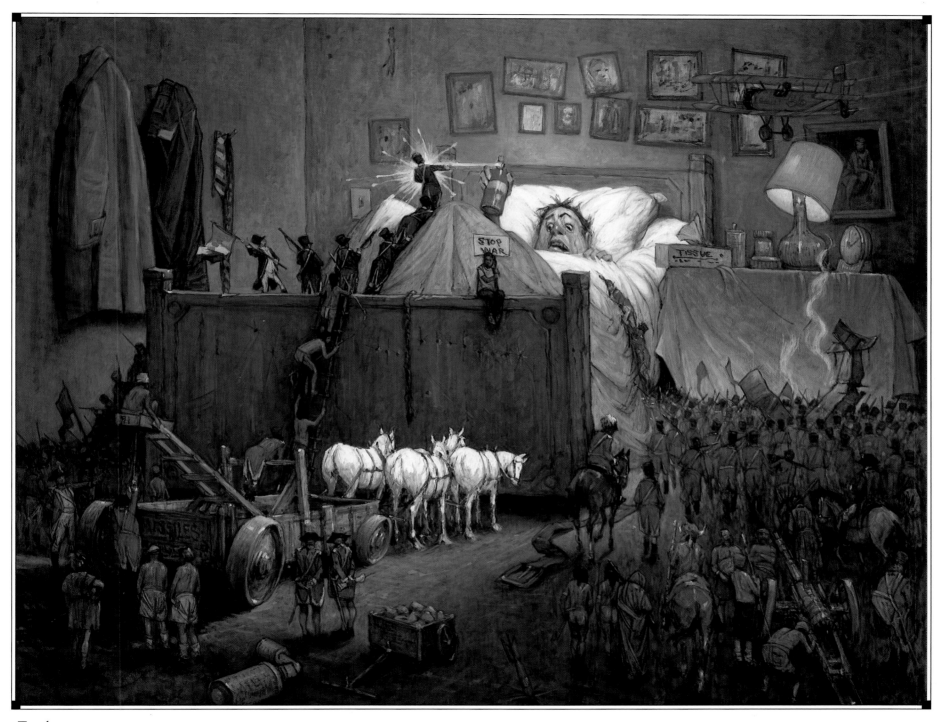

The Allergist – 24" x 30" (61.5cm x 77cm)

THE ALTERNATIVE PRACTITIONER

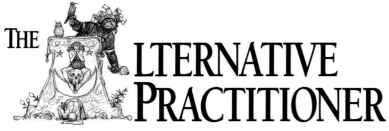

*A*lternative medicine is a recently popular, politically correct term that refers to all those methods of treatment which fall outside the blessing of conventional medicine. Mainstream medicine has lagged light-years behind its patients in recognizing the worth of many of these unconventional treatments. And practitioners have only recently been dragged, kicking and screaming, to the point of acknowledging their potential value.

This painting shows a rather healthy senior citizen who looks as if he could win his age group at the New York Marathon. He seems perfectly at ease as the numerous alternative practitioners minister to his needs. Acupuncture, biofeedback, vitamin therapy, reflexology, visualization, homeopathy, divine intervention, meditation, and therapeutic touch are all part of this canvas scene, just as they are a part of our world of medicine, from Zaire to Peking, from Paris to New York.

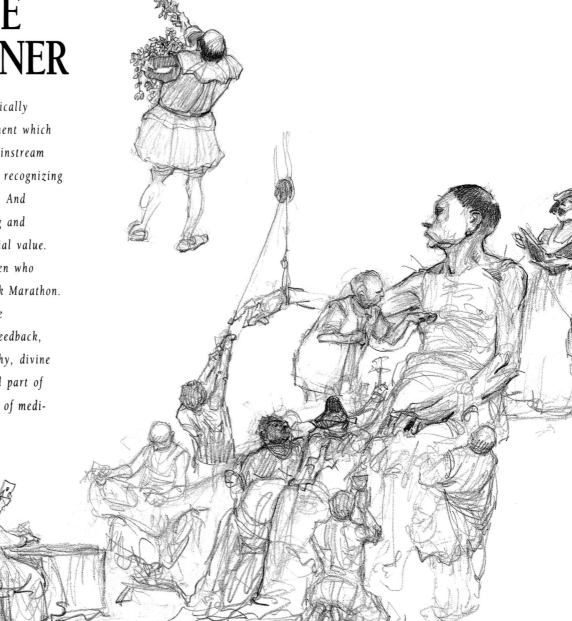

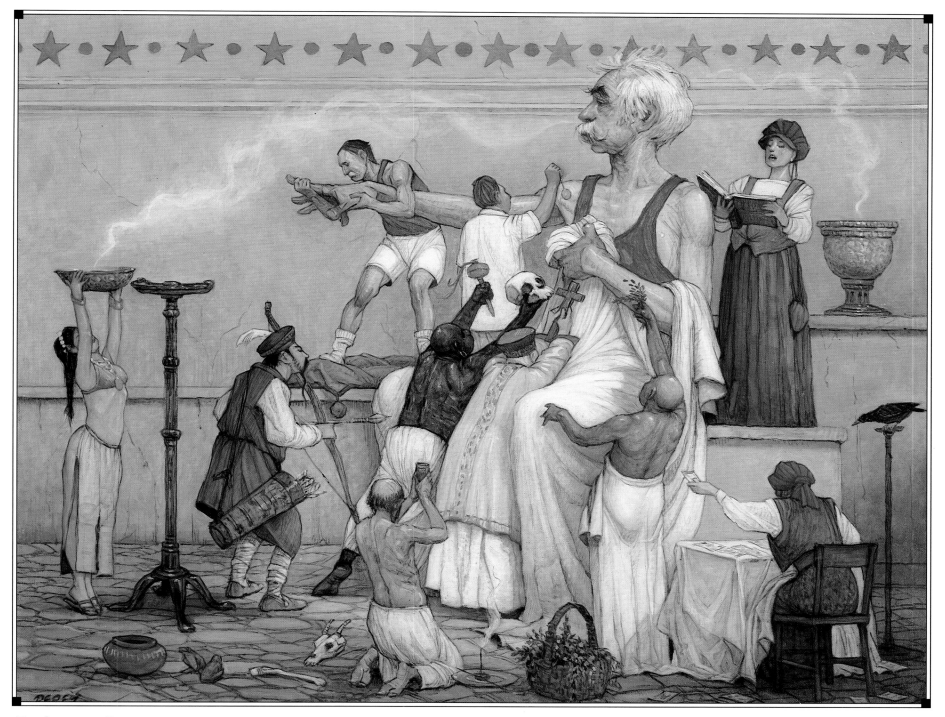

The Alternative Practitioner – 24" x 30" (61.5cm x 77cm)

THE 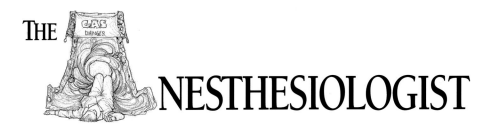NESTHESIOLOGIST

The anesthesiologist is often only a vaguely remembered actor from the surrealistic scenes that precede and follow surgery. With all the powers of Morpheus, the Greek god of sleep and dreams, the anesthesiologist seems to delight in his role as he smiles down on his vulnerable patient.

As the patient sleeps, the beautiful butterflies and horned devil become part of her mental confusion. Perhaps she dreams about which way her soul will go if she doesn't wake up again in this world.

In the meantime, her defenseless body will be handed over to the real "god" of the operating room, the surgeon.

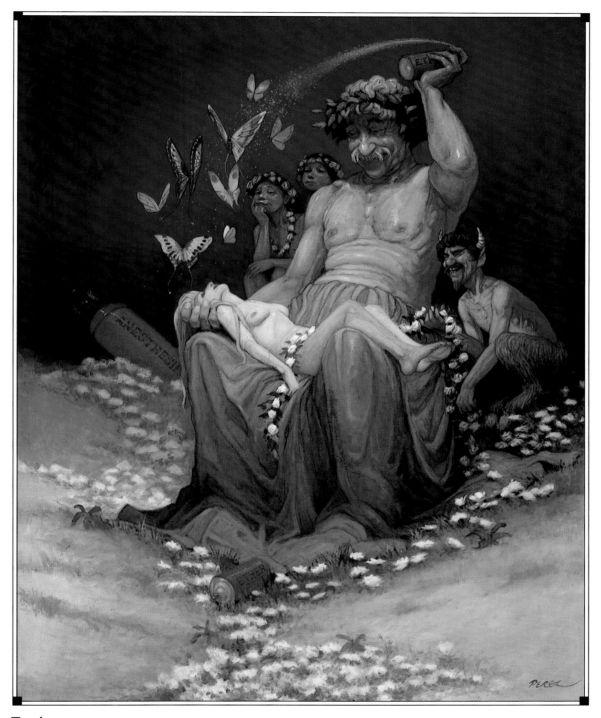

The Anesthesiologist – 24" x 30" (61.5cm x 77cm)

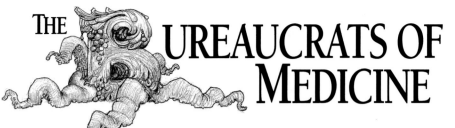

THE BUREAUCRATS OF MEDICINE

"The Bureaucrats of Medicine" is Perez' most politically correct painting in this series. Over twenty-five percent of U.S. health-care costs go toward pushing paper. Government workers, insurance reimbursers, social-care providers, legal eagles, accountants, record keepers, receptionists, secretaries, and the members of associations, societies, and foundations, make up a larger group than doctors, nurses, pharmacologists, and therapists combined. The bureaucratic tail is wagging our health-care dog.

Perez' satirical genius comes through at its best in the centrally placed, villainous puppeteer, a caricature of Dickens' Scrooge, impairing the doctor and manipulating the puppet patients. While the nurses are helplessly buried in paperwork, the bureaucrats in Washington are above it all and arrogantly toasting their own good health. The chap riding the paper airplane enjoys it all, and is not the least bit bothered by the salvage yard of patients or the environmental destruction behind him. He must be one of the ubiquitous third-party providers, pragmatically capable of adjusting to the changing winds of medical economics.

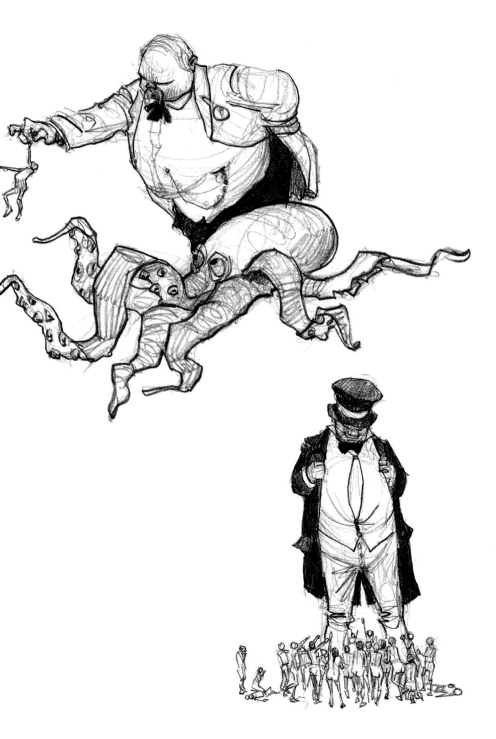

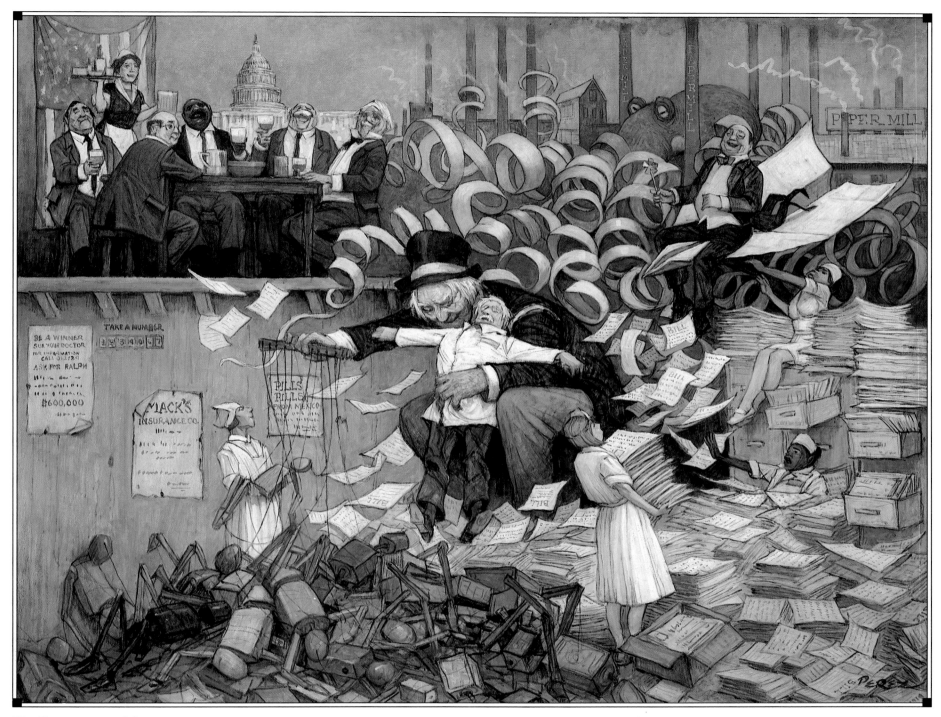

The Bureaucrats *of* Medicine *– 24" x 30" (61.5cm x 77cm)*

THE 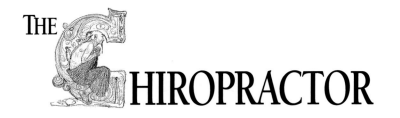HIROPRACTOR

This Doctor of Chiropractic, to keep up with his competitors, is broadcasting the successes of his treatments to anyone who will listen. The skeleton is the teaching tool that reminds us of the many problems resulting from our evolutionary predilection for standing upright instead of crouching on all fours.

The Buddhist caressing the patient's hand symbolizes the importance of touching to this profession. The patient seems quite relaxed as her legs are manipulated and an adjustment to her spinal column is about to be done. Maybe she won't be quite as relaxed when the fellow with the mallet steps in for a little percussion massage.

The earthen jugs symbolize the assimilation of holistic medicine and nutritional supplements into the mainstream of chiropractic. What is in them, nobody knows—but this patient seems to be thriving.

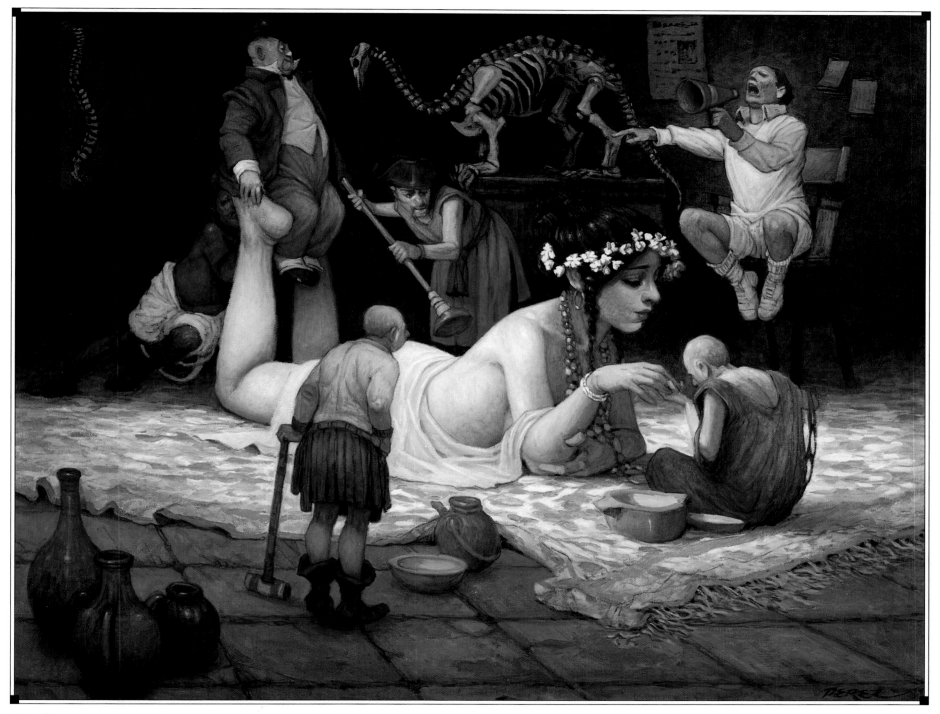

The Chiropractor – 24" x 30" (61.5cm x 77cm)

THE DENTIST

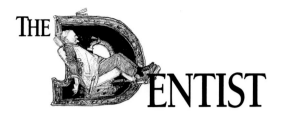

Remember the old childhood joke? "How does a dentist examine an alligator's teeth? Very carefully!" Well, the dentist in this painting obviously doesn't remember it. In fact, he is performing his examination on the patient's turf rather than on his own. This might be much nicer for all patients than lying in the dentist's chair with eyes tightly closed to shut out memories of past ordeals.

The wart hog with the spittoon, the fat fellow prying open the jaws, and the doctor with his head buried in the patient's mouth, fit well with the distortions of reality induced by whiffs of nitrous oxide. Of course, no one really laughs in the dental chair, and here even the monkey seems serious, while the doctor's nurse stoically records the locations of the newly discovered caries.

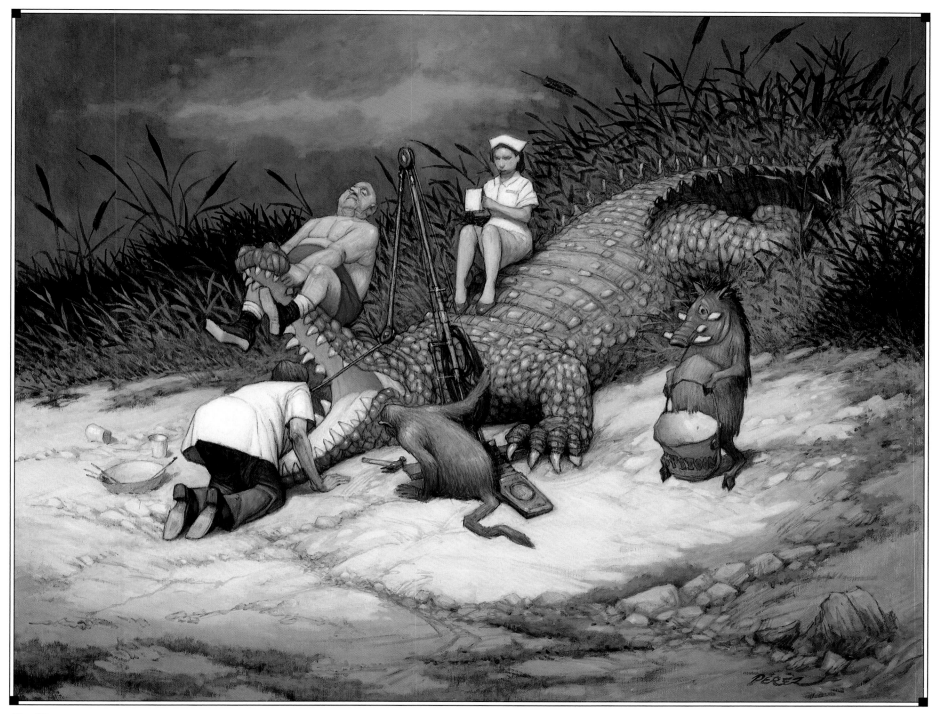

The Dentist – 24" x 30" (61.5cm x 77cm)

THE 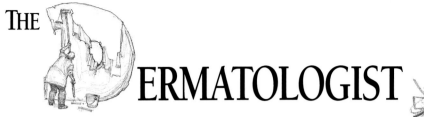ERMATOLOGIST

Doctors like to say that dermatology is the perfect specialty, since "patients never get well, never die, and never call at night." But if the dermatologist happens to be treating a tiger, all bets are off.

The magnificent tiger in this painting has gone to the doctor because he has lost his stripes. What could be more stressful to a tiger than this? His identity and ego are at stake. Who could restore his splendid coat more competently than a dermatologist?

The doctor and nurse in this painting seem to be approaching their needlework with due diligence and planning, but the audience of monkeys seems unimpressed. Maybe they know from experience that, if for any reason the doctor inadvertently sticks the patient, or, heaven forbid, the transplanted stripes are rejected, this placid tiger may suddenly rouse and have the doctor and his staff for lunch. What a metaphor of a malpractice suit!

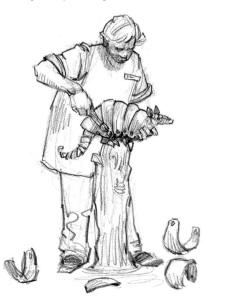

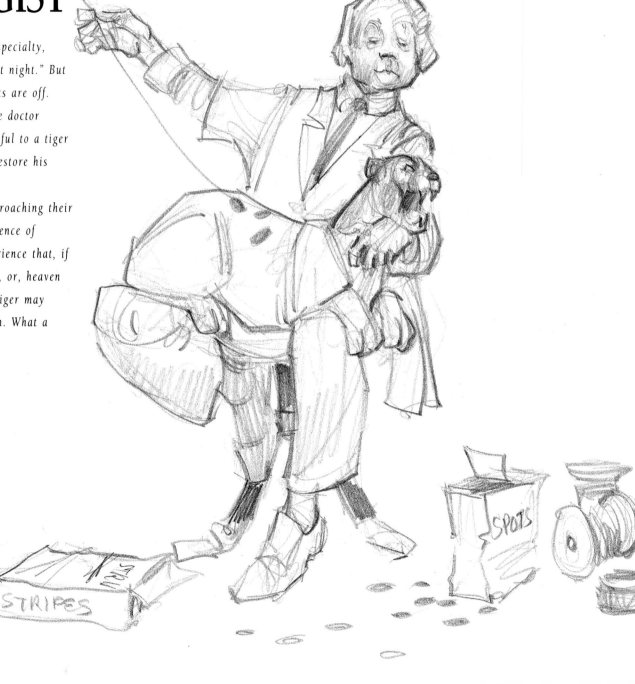

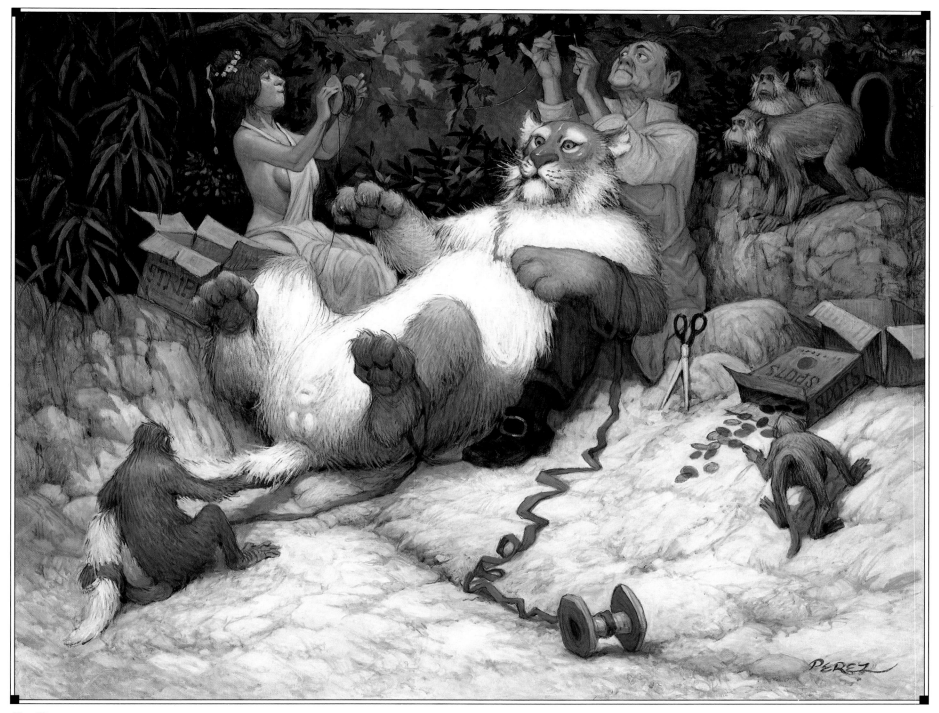

The Dermatologist – 24" x 30" (61.5cm x 77cm)

THE 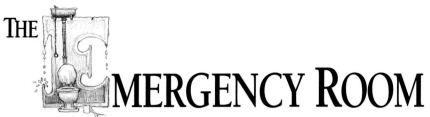MERGENCY ROOM

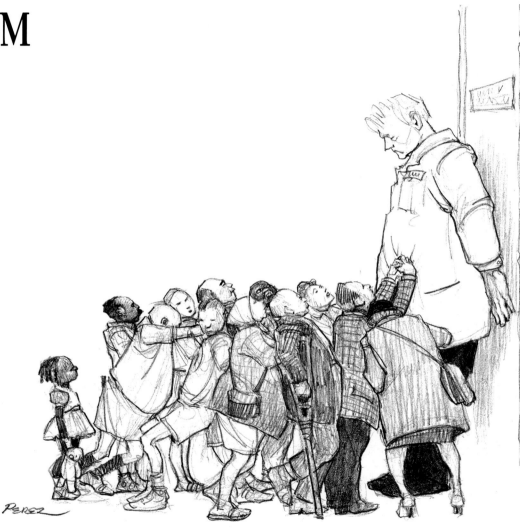

While planning this painting, Perez spent a night at a large city hospital emergency room and was reminded of the night he and his wife had taken his ill grandson to the ER. There, Perez and his wife found a long line of people waiting to be cared for, with nowhere else to go for treatment. Although most of the crowd waited patiently, one old man grew tired of waiting and decided to do something about it. He stretched himself out in the middle of the floor, pretending to be near death. Immediately, two men came with a stretcher, picked the old fellow up, and hauled him into an examining room.

In his painting, Perez has the members of the medical staff towering over the crowd of diminutive patients, symbolizing the sometimes intimidating nature of today's hospitals. While death waits in the form of a vulture perched atop the stoplight, the TV cameraman tries to catch a little drama for the eleven o'clock news.

The lame, the blind, the pregnant, and the sick migrate endlessly to the center of the canvas, where they are unceremoniously shoveled onto the examining table like pieces of coal into a furnace, with no privacy or sanctity.

While the antique ambulance is a reminder of the days of World War I, the contemporary posters on the wall bring today's health-education efforts into view. The policeman tries to stop the flow of patients. As the street vendor displays her wares, she views the scene and, like so many of us, is glad she is only a spectator— at least for today.

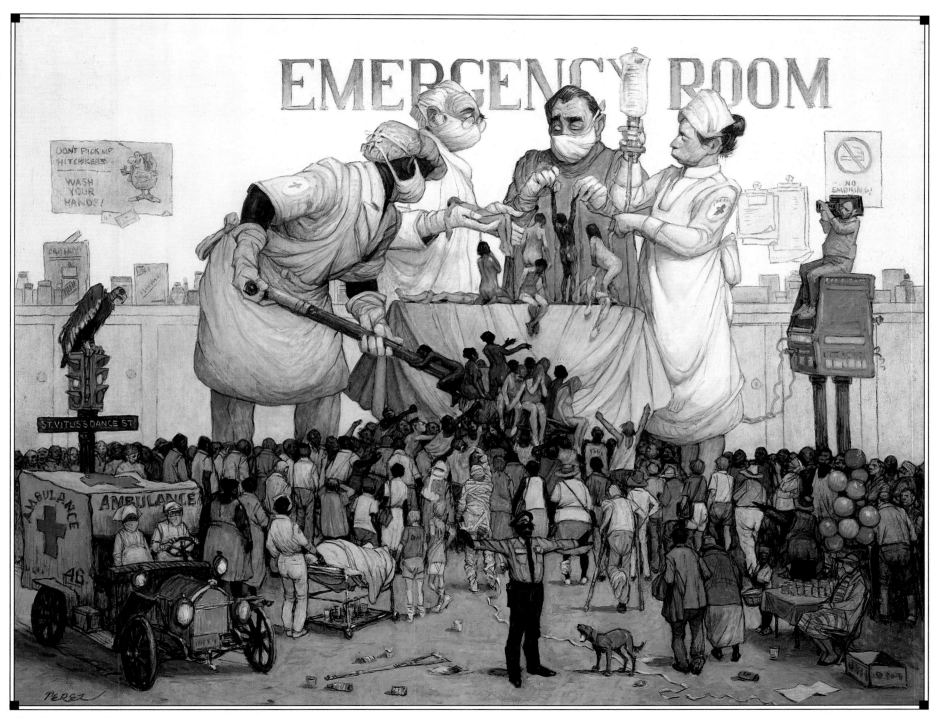

The Emergency Room – 24" x 30" (61.5cm x 77cm)

THE 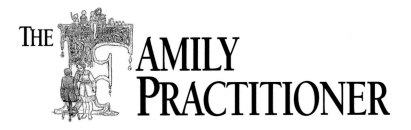AMILY PRACTITIONER

This painting reminds us that doctors are human, too. They get worn out and weary and succumb to the same stresses as their patients. This poor family "doc" is like the old woman who lived in a shoe. He has so many patients he doesn't know what to do.

Since the doctor appears to be overcome by the demands of his practice, his assistant patiently offers him some of his own medicine. Meanwhile, the patients appear to be faring better than the doctor.

The small, malnourished black child and the undernourished white child swinging on the rope are symbols of world hunger. The crying, naked child held by the mother in shorts, and the lady with the deaf old man tell us that most of us will be as children twice.

The man sitting on the doctor's knee nonchalantly reads the paper, exemplifying the ability of some people to remain detached, no matter what the impending diagnosis may be. The inebriated chap between the doctor's feet shows another way of coping with examining-room anxiety.

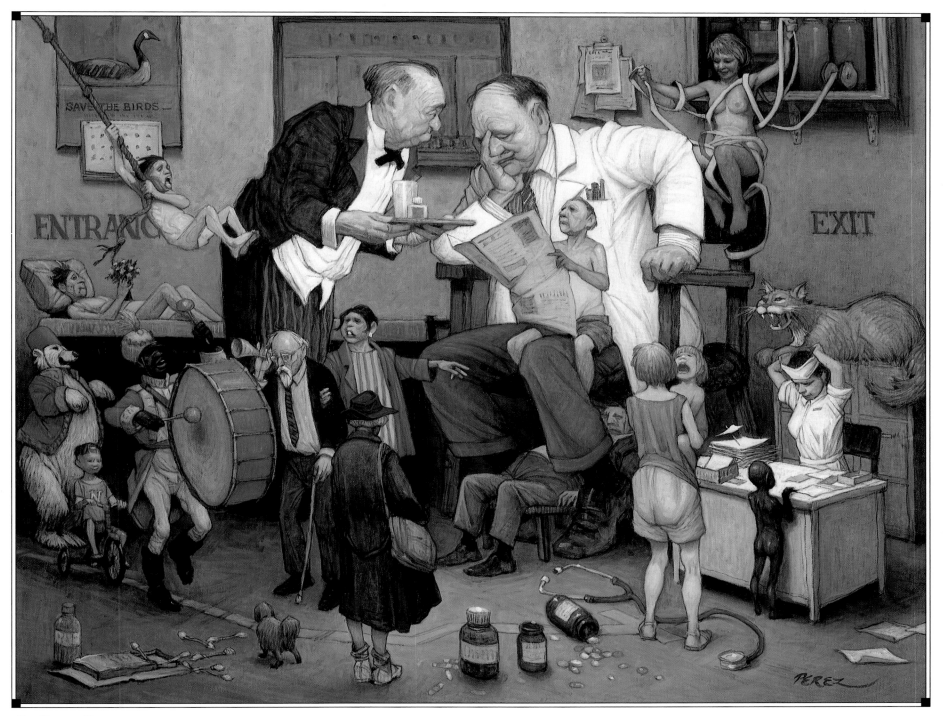

The Family Practitioner – 24" x 30" (61.5cm x 77cm)

THE 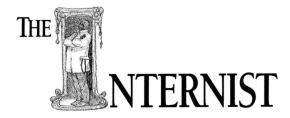NTERNIST

*T*he medieval setting Perez chose for this painting seems to fit the personality of the specialty. It also adds strength to Perez' belief that men still hold archaic opinions about women and often treat them accordingly. Yet, when things go wrong, they often cry for their mother—hence the woman internist.

The churchmen and court attendants represent all the other professionals who surround the department of internal medicine—and there's a strong contingent from the area of religion. Is that because the internist needs divine direction, or because the patient may need to be helped into the next world?

In spite of the fact that he is symbolically larger than the doctor, the patient certainly dares not question her medical judgment. The assistants reverently participate in the ritual of the placing of the electrodes. Meanwhile, who or what is on the other side of the door? Could it be the hospital review committee, the only entity with the audacity to question a discharge diagnosis? Or could it be the all-powerful, third-party payer who will accept or reject the doctor's fees for services with the flick of a computer printout?

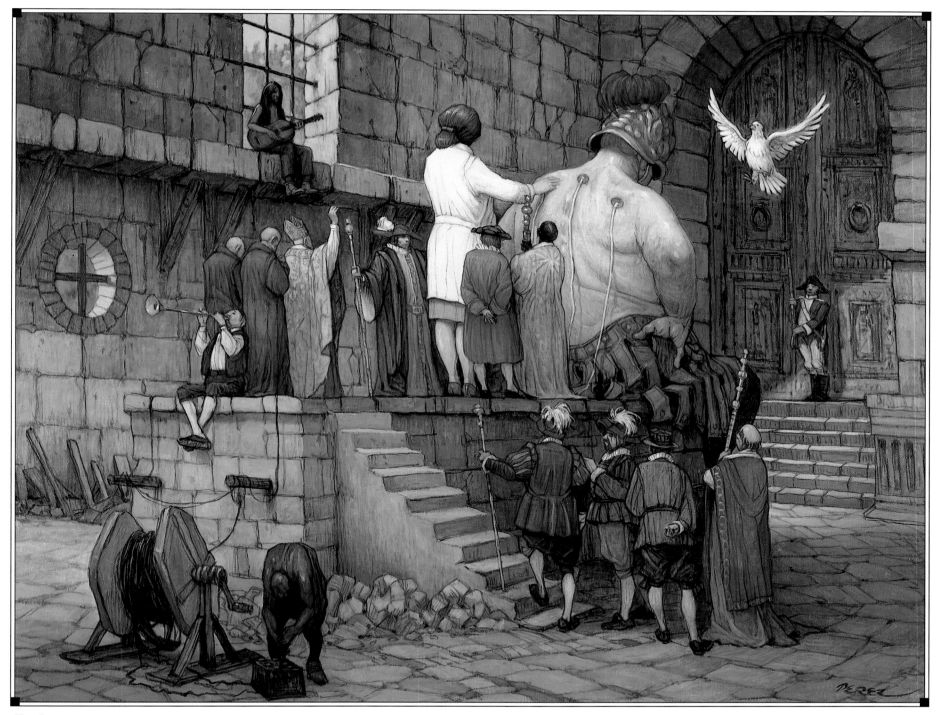

The Internist – 24" x 30" (61.5cm x 77cm)

THE 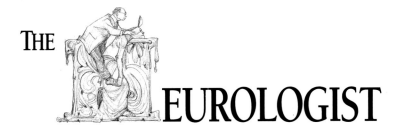EUROLOGIST

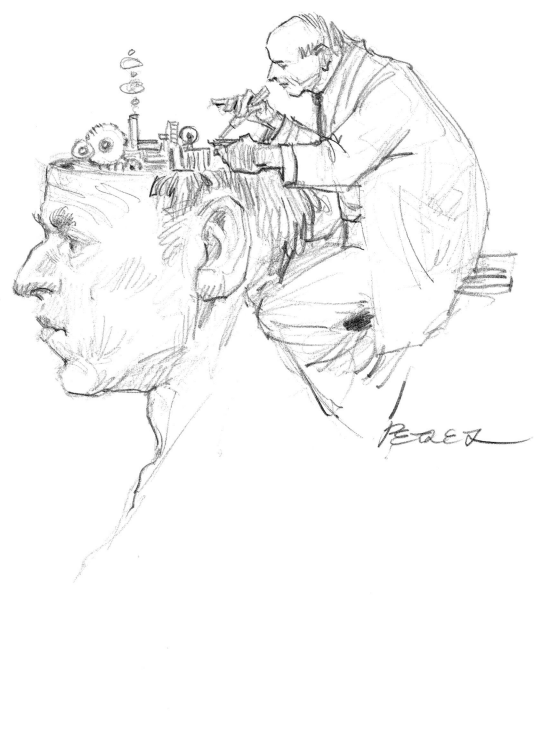

Neurologists love to observe and measure. Historically, their tools have been the percussion hammer for knee jerks, the vibrating fork for bone conduction, and the pins for determining whether the patient is numb or faking it. Today, neurologists use electroencephalograms to tell when we're brain dead.

Medical students can spot a neurology professor a ward away. They're almost invariably serious-minded, academically oriented males with a penchant for raising the possibility of an extremely rare and always incurable malady named after some seventeenth-century Frenchman. Polyneuropathy, neuroprexia, amyotrophia, and encephalopathy are just some of the hard-to-pronounce words neurologists typically love to let casually roll from their tongues. No doubt the doctor peering into the centaur's skull is about to pronounce the poor fool as suffering from anencephaly.

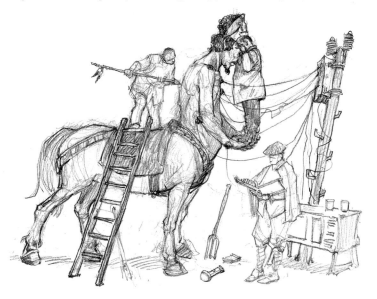

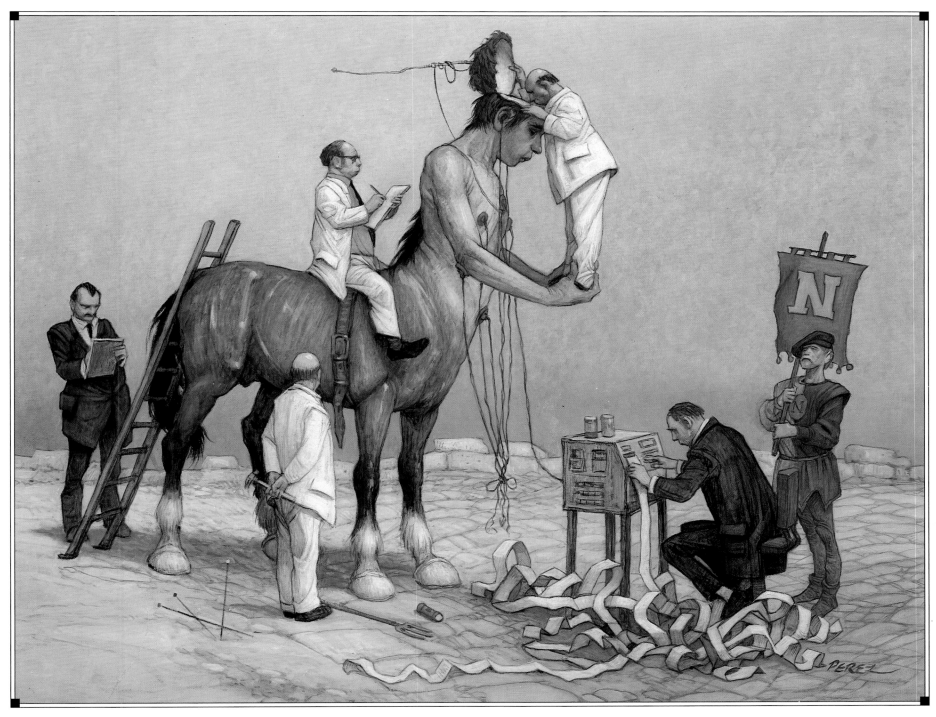

The Neurologist – 24" x 30" (61.5cm x 77cm)

THE 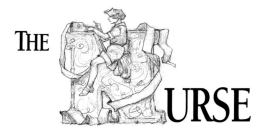URSE

Nursing has been defined as both art and science, Florence Nightingale having called it the finest of the arts. In this painting, Perez reinforces the notion that nursing is not merely a technique, but a process that incorporates the elements of soul, mind, and imagination.

Art, music, flowers, a Superman T-shirt—this patient is really "king for a day." But there's an extra-special reason for this treatment, because Perez has painted himself as the patient, even to the get-well card above the bed reading "Dear Jose."

Every art gallery has its nursing saints, nurturing mothers, healing miracles, sickbeds and lying-in chambers, but Perez has placed his nurses in a whimsical sickroom that symbolizes the child in all of us. He fondly remembers his "sick-in-bed" school days when he was pampered with all kind of special privileges. The piñata is from his childhood in Mexico, the crayons and coloring books show that his artistic talents also go back to those days, and the brushes in the lower left-hand corner make the transition from his childhood fantasies to his adult talents.

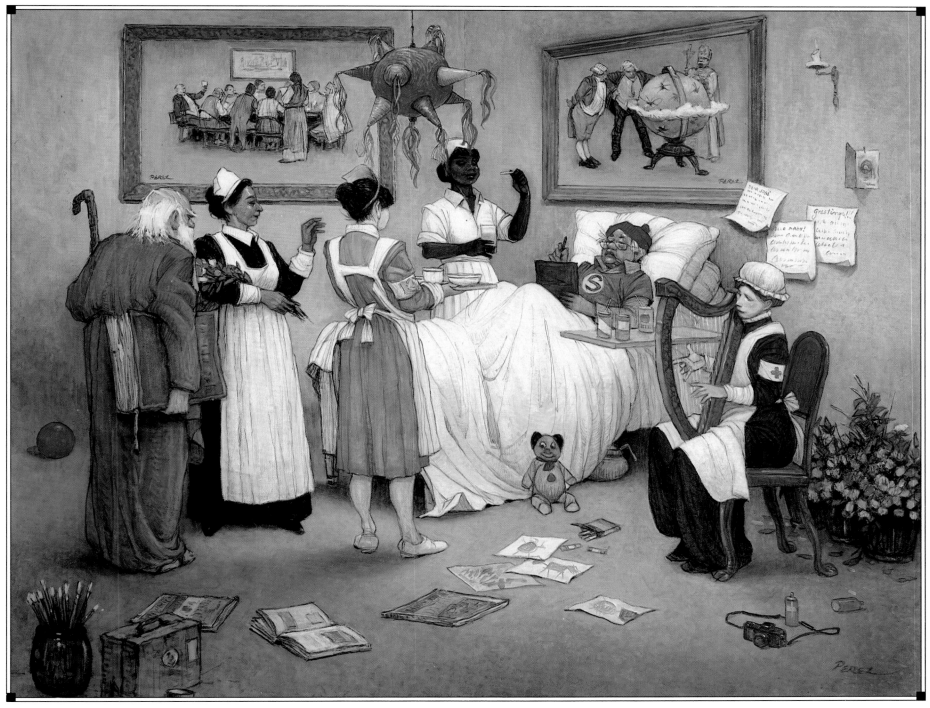

The Nurse – 24" x 30" (61.5cm x 77cm)

THE 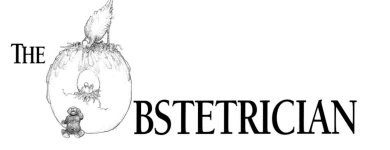BSTETRICIAN

Perez based this work on the supposition that an unborn baby inside its mother's womb can hear everything that's going on outside. If this is true, this baby was well-informed. Note that he offers a flag of surrender to the doctor, but, just in case things don't go well, he is prepared to fight him with a pop gun!

The instruments and toys of war that reflect our violent society form a striking contrast to the peaceful presence of the chicks and doves. The new mother, attended by little cherubs, seems to be blissfully preoccupied—perhaps with reading the latest advice on raising children successfully. The pregnant black girl patiently waits behind the doctor, her status revealed by her diminutive size. Notice the body language of the nurse. While she is only assisting, it looks as if she could take over as a midwife at a minute's notice.

What is the doctor handing the newborn—a bill, a card for his next appointment, or an official ID card welcoming him into the human race?

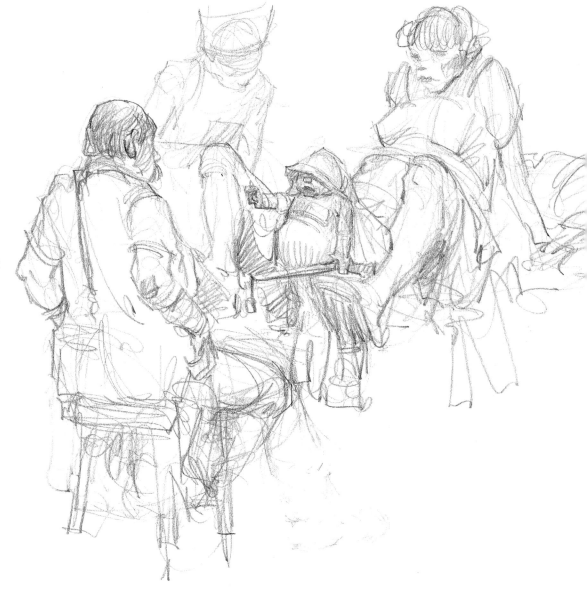

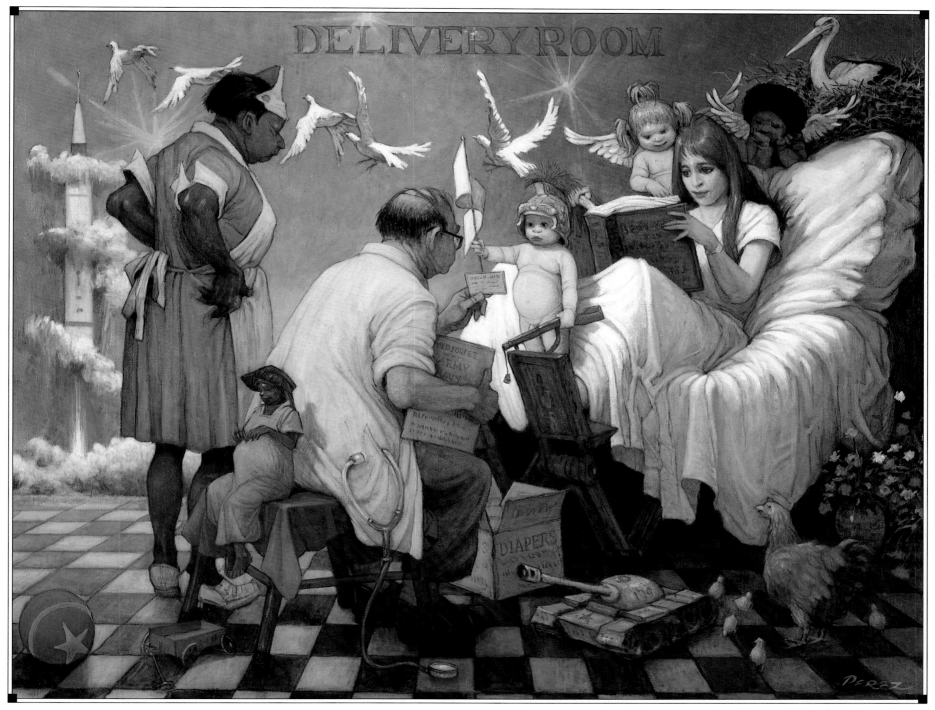

The Obstetrician – 24" x 30" (61.5cm x 77cm)

THE 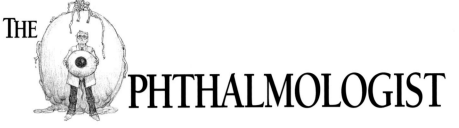OPHTHALMOLOGIST

Perez has a special appreciation for ophthalmologists because
he suffers from glaucoma. If it were not for eye surgery he would no
longer be painting. Perez knows firsthand what it is like to make
frequent visits to the eye doctor.

This doctor is a caricature of Perez' own doctor, and Perez is
the patient with the vision problems. Perez says, "I would bet ten
to one that the unorthodox practices of this doctor's test for color
blindness (redhead or blonde?) would make most any chap's eyes pop
like corks on champagne bottles and see anew."

Other parts of this painting show
unexplained subplots and all sorts
of ingenious ways to test the
eyes that would do justice to the
original Rube Goldberg.

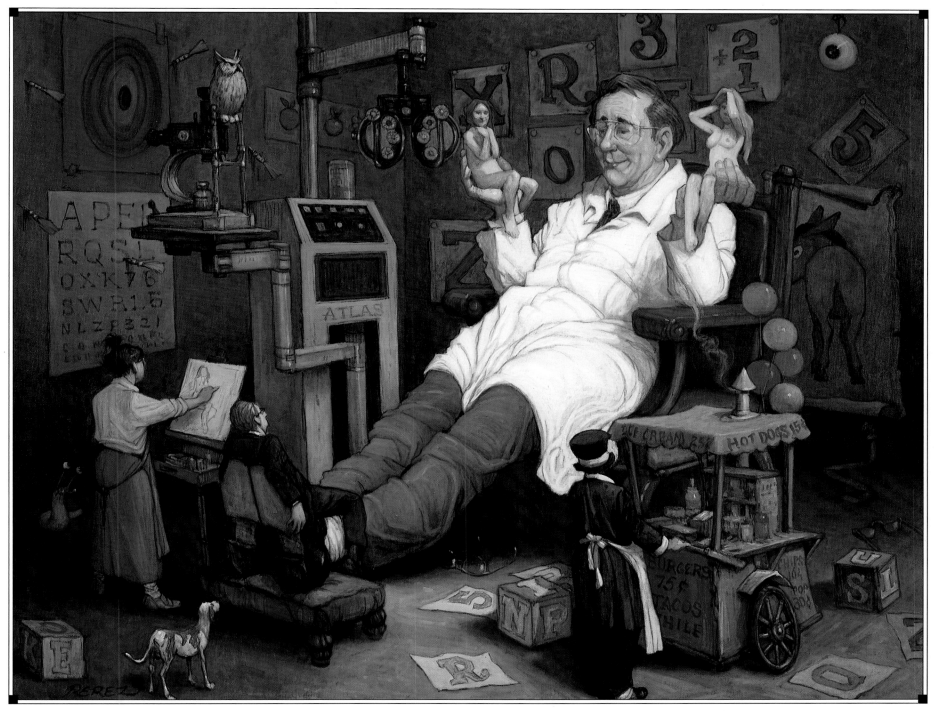

The Ophthalmologist – 24" x 30" (61.5cm x 77cm)

THE 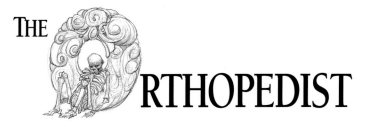RTHOPEDIST

A gargantuan figure, the doctor in this painting sits on his
unique throne of bones and conveys a sense of power and authority.
The ruins of the Roman wall and the Egyptian nurse standing in front
of the doctor are signs that orthopedics is one of the oldest branches
of medicine. In fact, archaeologists and paleontologists have found
evidence of set bones dating back to primitive times.

Various athletes approach the doctor's throne to ask in
reverential fashion for healing of their sports injuries. They
probably already know that complete obedience to the doctor's
commands will be demanded of them. The doctor will surely tell
them to stop doing whatever they are doing, or, if they're not
doing something, to begin it.

The enormous size accorded the doctor could reflect the fact
that many orthopedists played football in their college days and
still enjoy being on the sidelines in their role as doctors. Or it
could simply be acknowledgment of the degree of trust
placed in him by his patients, who are probably the
most compliant of patients because of
their desire to return to their sport
as soon as possible.

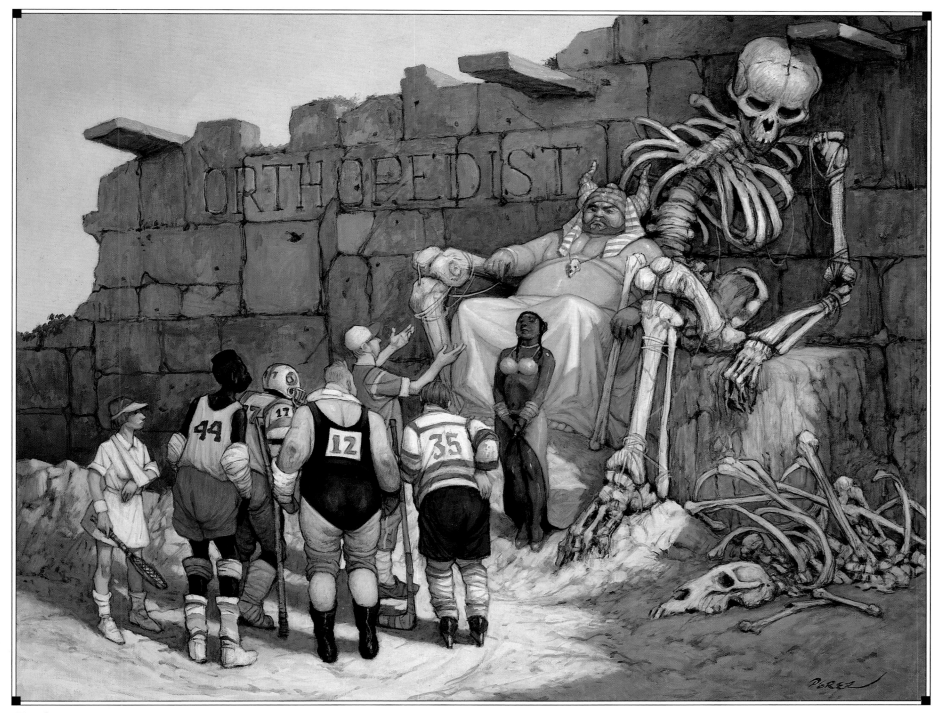

The Orthopedist – 24" x 30" (61.5cm x 77cm)

THE 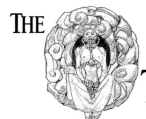 OTORHINOLARYNGOLOGIST

*I*magine *the challenge of treating this patient for a nosebleed, chronic rhinitis, or a blocked eustachian tube! What better patient for the ear, nose, and throat doctor than an elephant? These otorhinolaryngologists could spend hours trying out all their latest fiber-optic scopes on this patient's elongated nose. And what a playground these ears make for one fascinated by external canals and tympanic membranes! Imagine removing a ball of wax from these caverns.*

Although this patient looks cooperative and docile, the doctor must never forget that a sneeze might be disastrous. And if the assistant happens to step on a ticklish toe, it might provoke an uproarious protest and result in one squashed assistant.

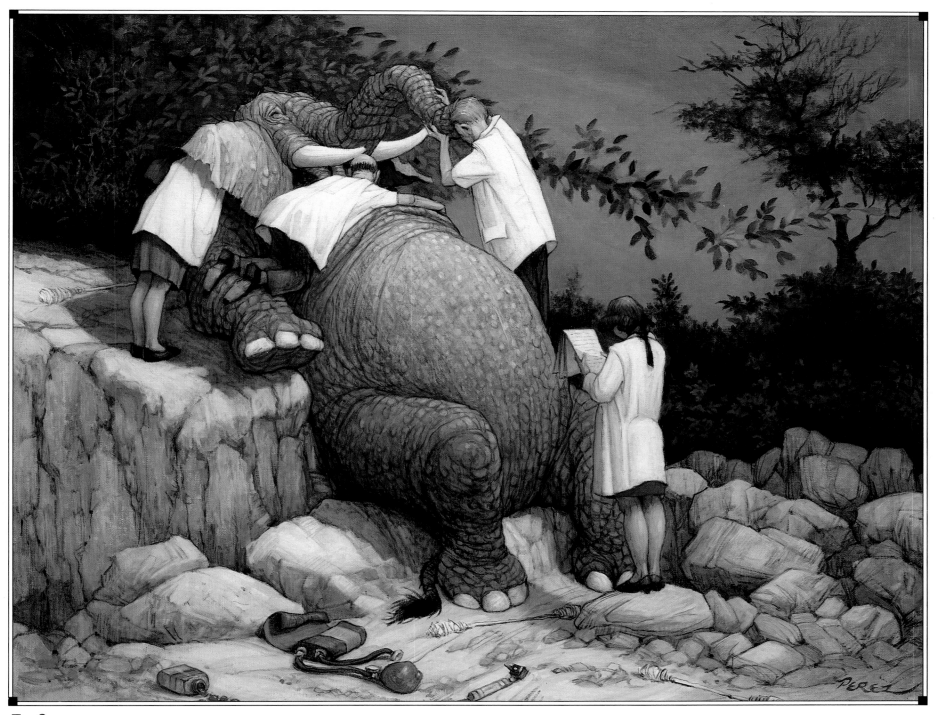

The Otorhinolaryngologist – 24" x 30" (61.5cm x 77cm)

THE PATHOLOGIST

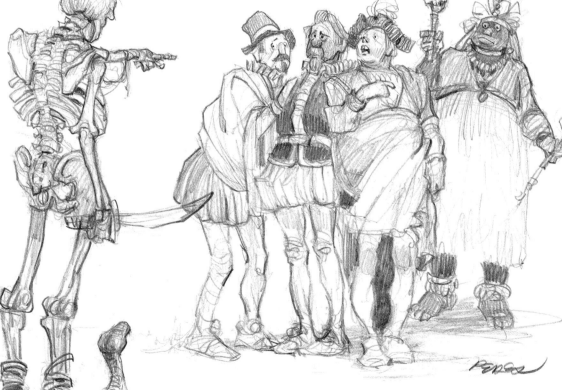

*T*he pathologist usually has the last word in medicine, because he does the autopsy. He tells everyone else what the correct diagnosis should have been and why the treatments didn't work. He can also be the ace in the hole for a malpractice defense attorney, and the secret weapon of the plaintiff's attorney.

In this painting, the tables seem to have been turned on the pathologist. Death has come back to tell the pathologist what was done incorrectly. As Death straddles the Jungian snake amid a horde of rats on the morgue floor—symbolic of the carriers of the disease that caused the plagues of earlier times—he points an accusatory finger at the doctor and his assistants.

The assistants may know about many more mistakes, judging from their fears of the defiant skeleton. Even the witch doctor looks a little frazzled as he tries to use his magic to shift the blame to someone else.

Notice the autopsy knife, which the pathologist has dropped on the floor in fright. What fresh mistakes have been made on the body on the morgue table? Is the pathologist trying to bring this fellow back to life with all those strange contraptions? Is this what Death is chiding him about?

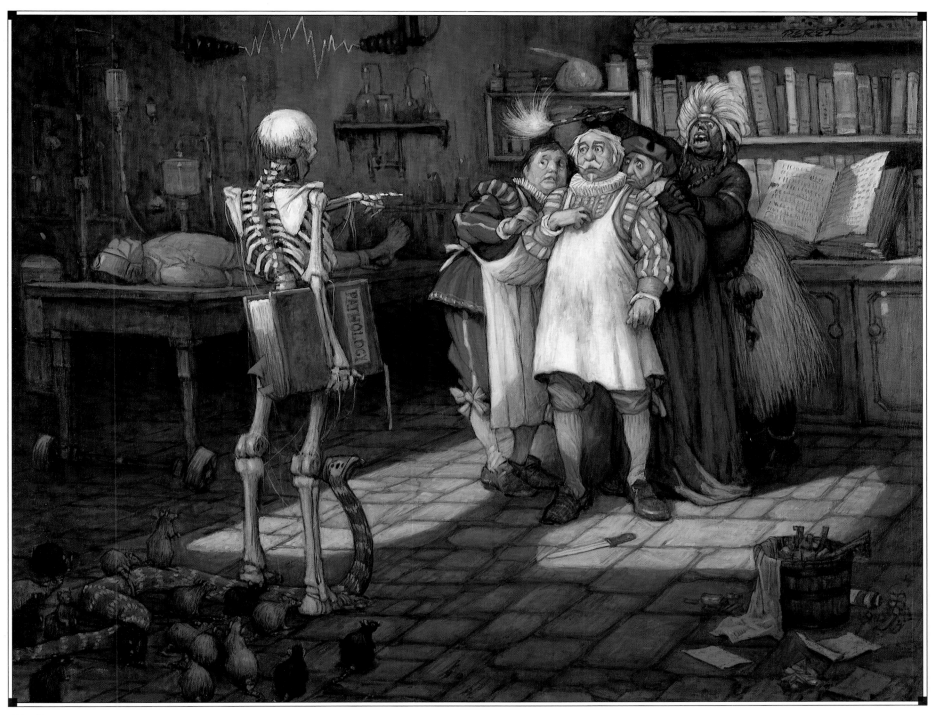

The Pathologist – 24" x 30" (61.5cm x 77cm)

THE 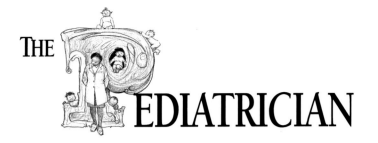PEDIATRICIAN

Perez painfully remembers his childhood days during the Depression, when there was little money for medical care. He is thankful for the care he was able to provide in later years for his own two daughters.

From a psychological standpoint, it's interesting to note that there are no sick children in this painting. Under the supervision of a mothering pediatrician, the little patients all seem to be enjoying healthy lives. And from the heavenly clouds, the babies yet to be born seem anxious to receive their first medical checkups.

It's a shame the Utopian happiness of this painting isn't a reality in our society today: Drugs, violence, and child abuse are all too real. But somehow, with regard to children, Perez wanted to show things the way they should be, not the way they often are.

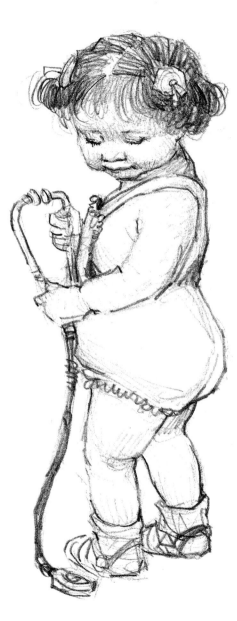

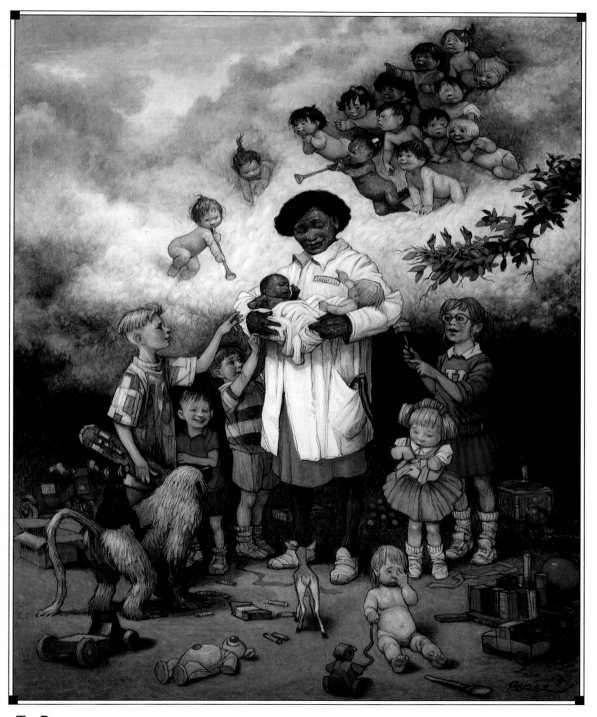

The Pediatrician – 30" x 24" (77cm x 61.5cm)

THE 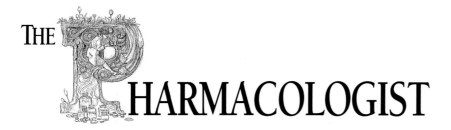HARMACOLOGIST

An adventurous chap and his assistant are out looking for exotic plants and butterflies in the hope of discovering new drugs. From the looks of the imps and the native girl, the woods are chock full of undiscovered pharmaceuticals.

The exploring pharmacologist seems to approach with glee the task of preparing his findings for study. He probably can't wait to write his observations in his daily journal. One can only guess what miracle psychotropic drugs may come from his discoveries.

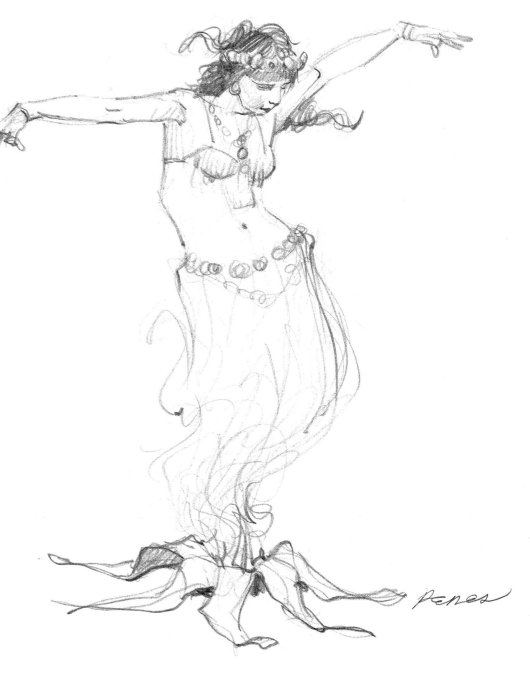

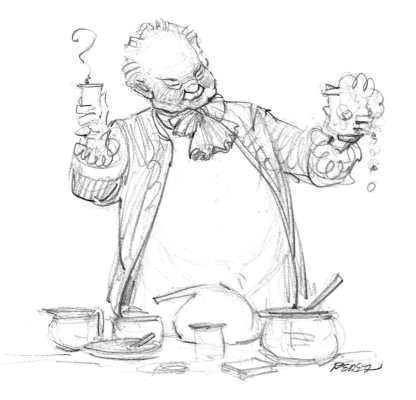

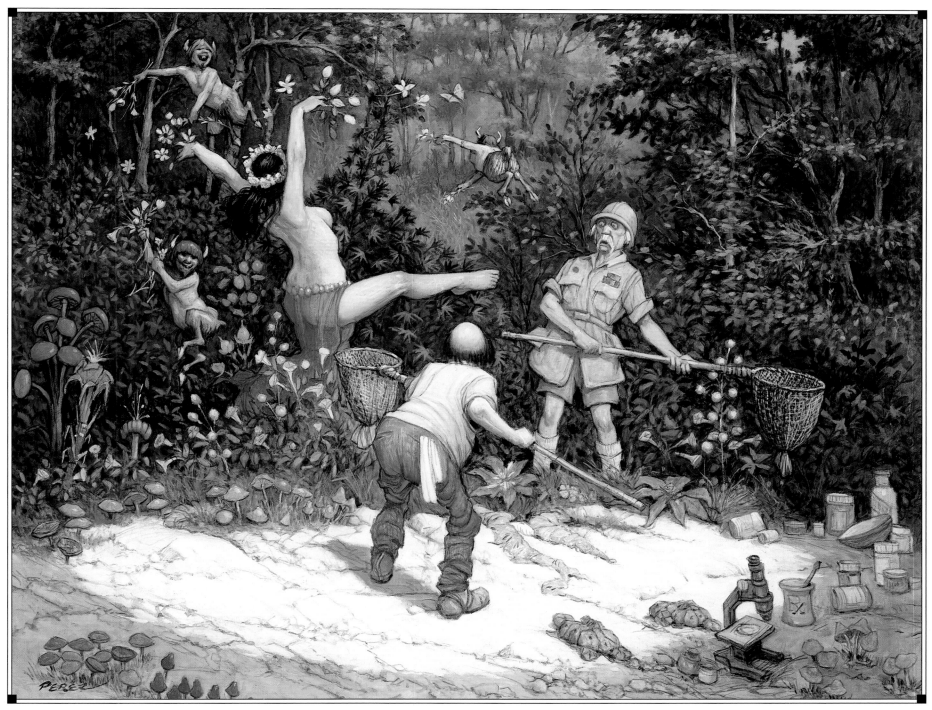

The Pharmacologist – 24" x 30" (61.5cm x 77cm)

THE PLASTIC SURGEON

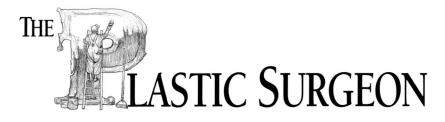

*S*ociety magazines often advertise the fountain of youth promised by plastic surgery, sometimes complete with payment plans and free consultations. To those for whom elective surgery is an option, these promises are often delivered. For those who need reconstructive or therapeutic surgery, the plastic surgeon is a lifeline.

Perez, however, has chosen to satirize those who expect elective miracles. His rotund doctor is half sculptor and half painter, whose patient believes he can turn an old lady into a young model. Similarly, the watchful toad expects to become a prince, the armadillo wants his skin to be as smooth as silk, and Frankenstein longs to look like a beach boy.

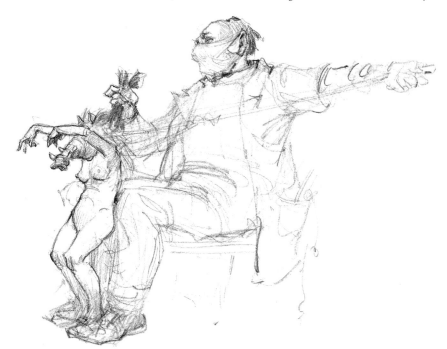

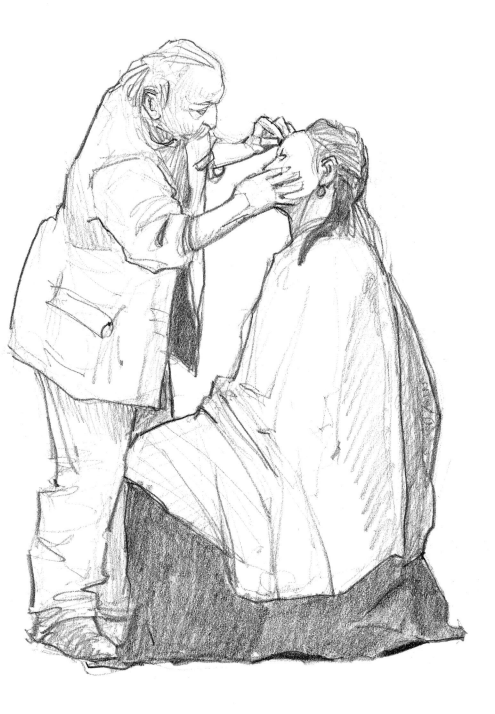

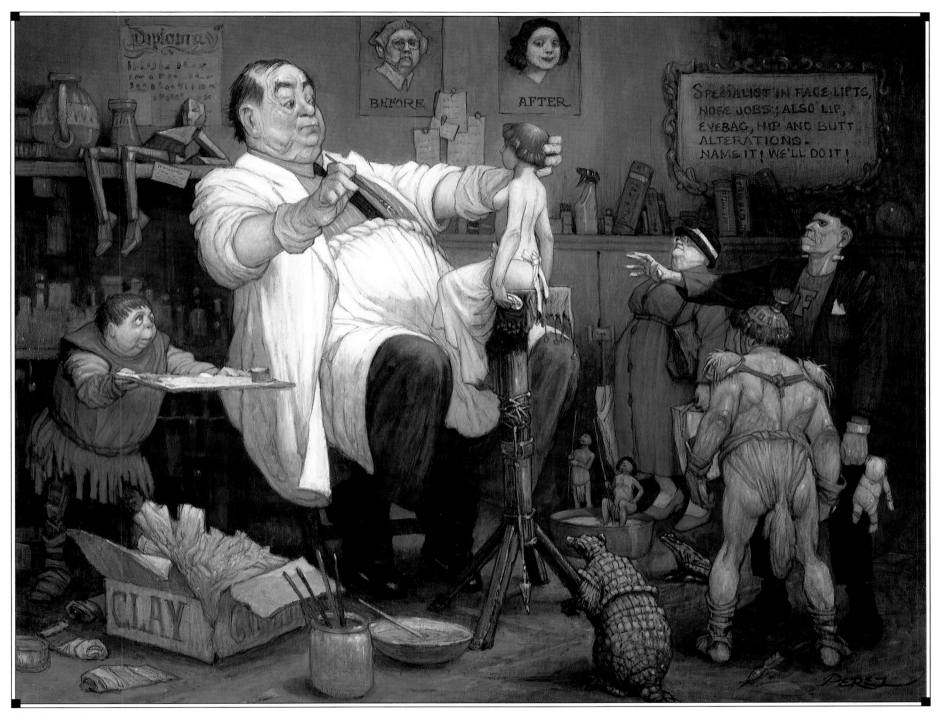

The Plastic Surgeon – 24" x 30" (61.5cm x 77cm)

THE 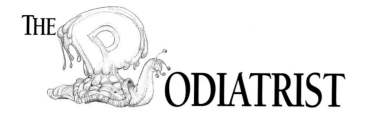ODIATRIST

Going to see a podiatrist is not nearly as frightening as going to a proctologist or a urologist. Few cancers occur on the feet, and most of the treatments are painless, so this patient is staying perfectly relaxed as the doctor and his assistants go about their business.

The full moon and stark landscape signify that the doctor doesn't need too many fancy tools to practice podiatry. No CAT scans, MRIs, or EKGs are necessary, only a few knives, files, and scissors, and enough common sense to know when to stop clipping away.

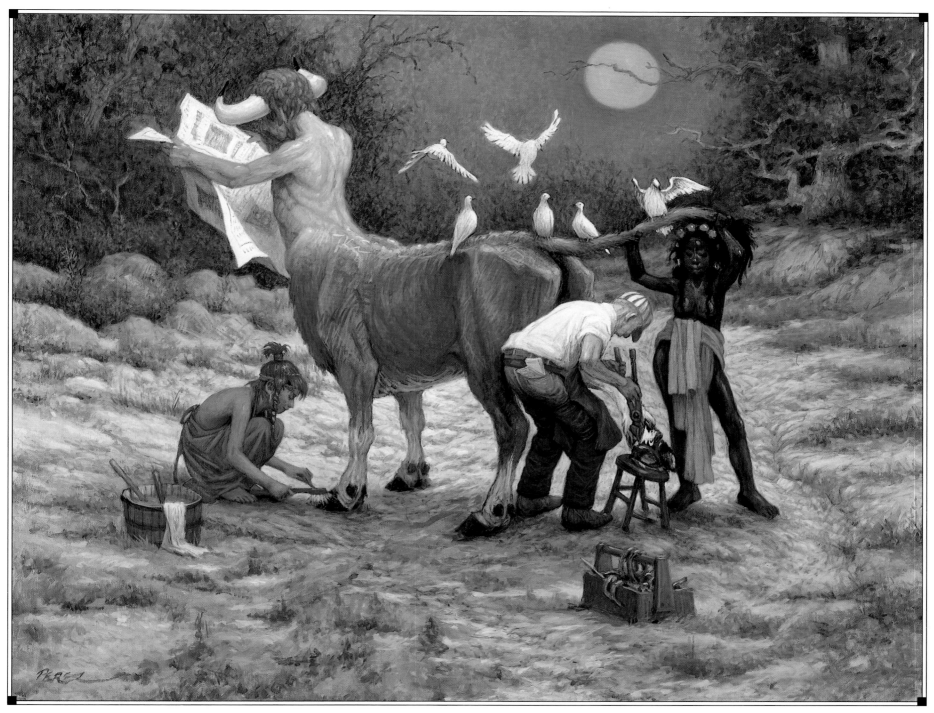

The Podiatrist – 24" x 30" (61.5cm x 77cm)

THE 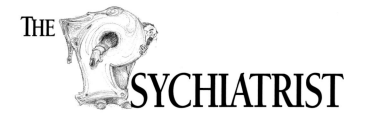SYCHIATRIST

This is the first painting Perez did for this collection, and it set the stage for the mind games he would play with each specialty. While a psychiatrist is supposed to be thinking about a patient's case, the psychiatrist in Perez' work is preoccupied with his own problems: His mistress is playing with his hair while illusions and delusions fill the room. Napoleon is there, with both arms shown in an uncharacteristic stance and a large Number One on his back. An anthropomorphic parrot awaits his turn to talk, a monkey is climbing on or off the doctor's back, an egg waits to hatch or be stepped on, and a dragon seems poised to strike. Trumpet sounds fill the air near the doctor's ear, and the drunken gladiator doesn't seem to know where to begin as he tells the doctor his troubles.

It's interesting to note the shoes on the psychiatrist. Is it significant that they are untied, or that they are running shoes?

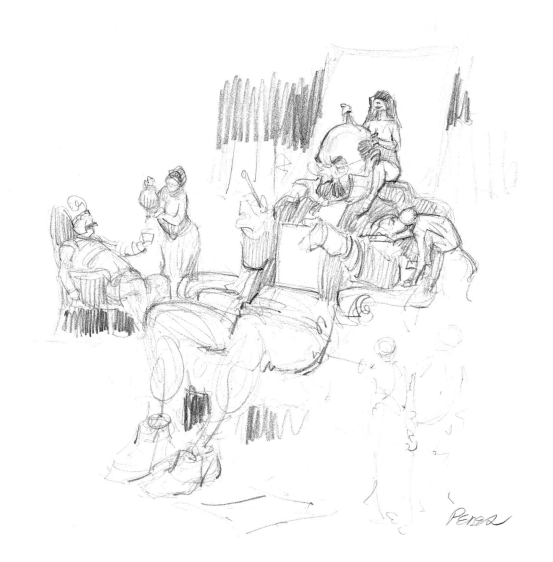

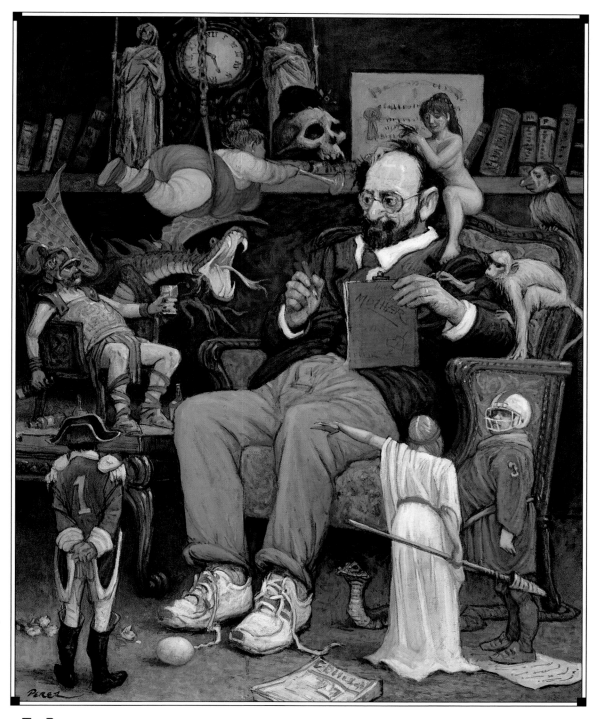

*T*he *P*sychiatrist – 30" x 24" *(77cm x 61.5cm)*

THE 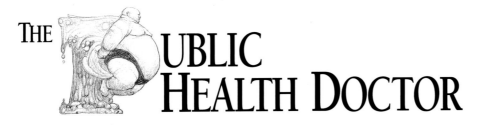UBLIC HEALTH DOCTOR

While surgeons, oncologists and radiologists symbolize modern medicine's infatuation with high-tech equipment, the field of public health medicine still deals principally with down-to-earth problems such as pollution, gun control, substance abuse, poor nutrition, bigotry, and superstition. Our sanitary engineers literally save more lives than our surgeons. When it comes to health, as Pogo said, "We have met the enemy, and the enemy is us."

This is the only painting in the series wherein Perez caricatures a recognizable, well-known doctor—former U.S. Surgeon General, C. Everett Koop. Dr. Koop receives this honor because Perez has been so impressed by Koop's leadership in national and global public health. God bless our unheralded public-health doctors.

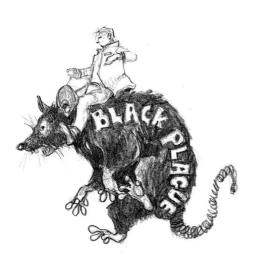

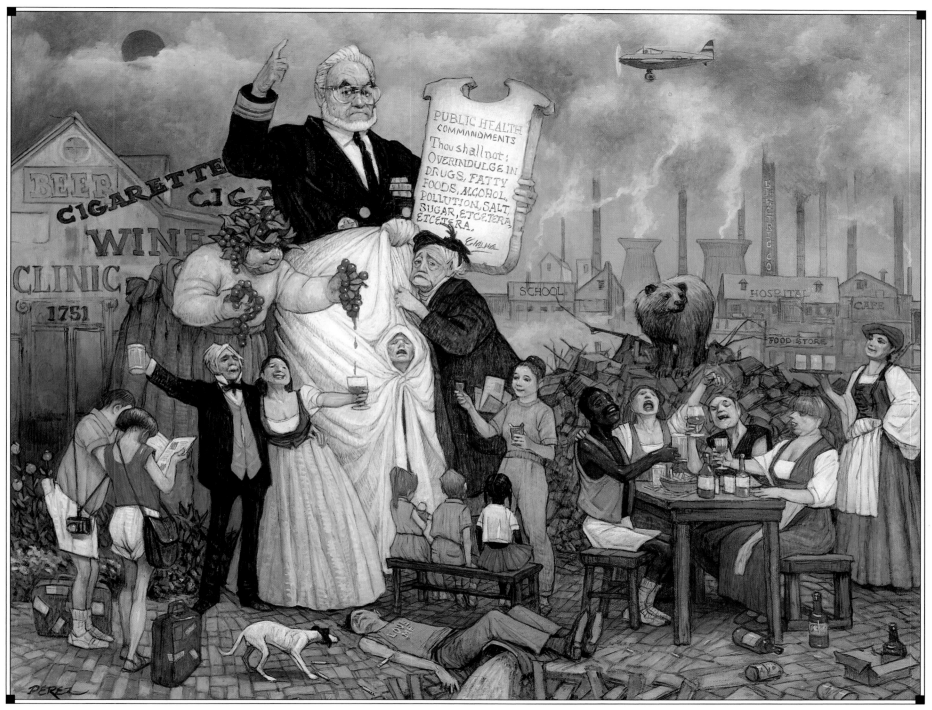

The Public Health Doctor – 24" x 30" (61.5cm x 77cm)

THE ~~X-RAYS~~ RADIOLOGIST

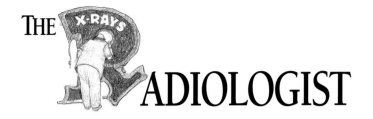

Appropriately enough, the painting of the radiologist is mostly in black and white. But it's also a relatively simple scene, which is ironic because X-ray medicine has probably become more high-tech than any other field of medicine.

Notice the body language of the two figures in this painting. The doctor seems to intuitively sense that she should keep her explanation as simple as possible as she tells her little patient what's going on in her skeleton. The clutch that the patient has on her doctor—and her dependence on the doctor's skill—is not returned by the doctor, who has her right arm awkwardly behind her back, instead of around the patient.

Perhaps Perez is trying to tell the viewer that, because radiologists often see very bad things going on inside the body before they are visible on the outside, they have a hard time letting themselves get close to their patients.

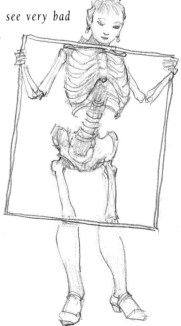

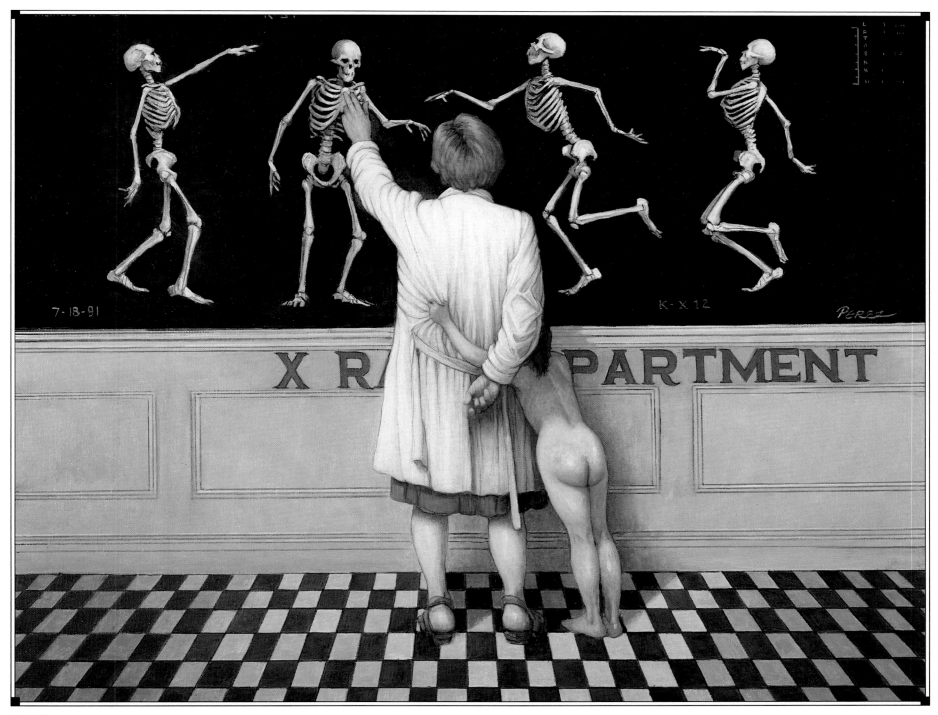

The Radiologist – 24" x 30" (61.5cm x 77cm)

THE SURGEON

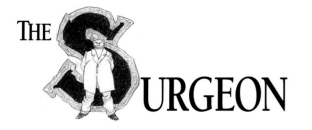

Although it may remind one of a repair shop, the operating room goes far beyond that. It represents the incredible innovations in medicine that have allowed man to repair and replace body parts. Someday we might be able to keep human beings running indefinitely, rather like restored antique cars.

Perez' block-and-tackle rig is testimony to the inestimable value of practical tools in even the most complicated of technical situations. It's somewhat reminiscent of one of those television scenes in which a white-coated doctor comes dashing out of a helicopter carrying a donor heart in a polystyrene drink cooler.

The size of the patient in relation to the size of the repairmen—the surgeons—is an interesting feature of this painting, perhaps to express the intricacy of the human body.

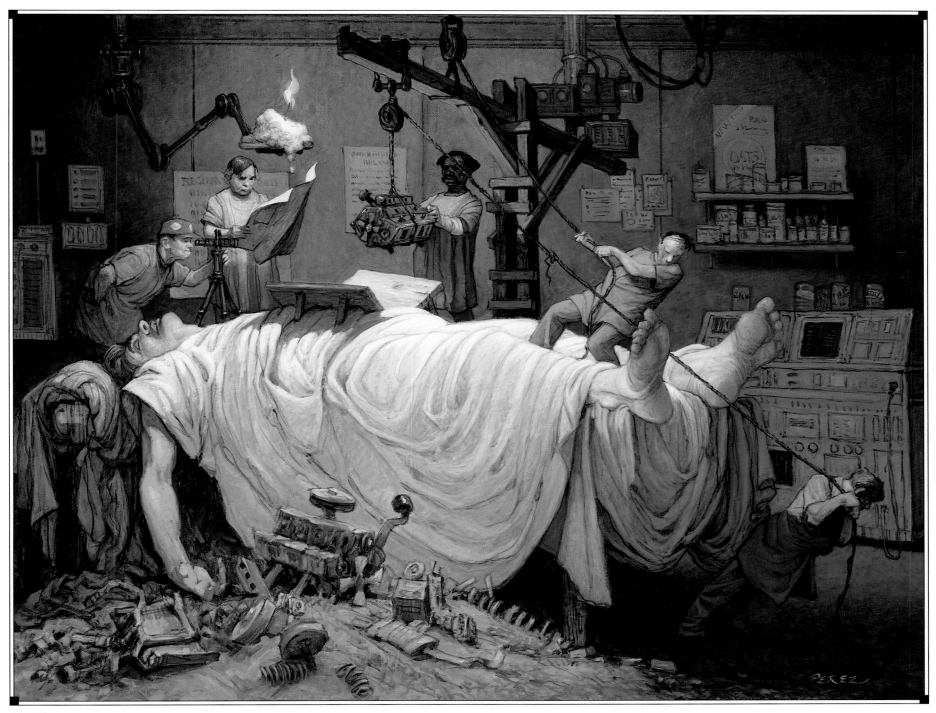

The Surgeon – 24" x 30" (61.5cm x 77cm)

THE 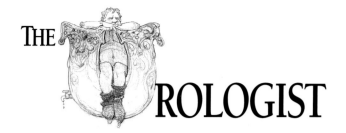ROLOGIST

The body language of the patient in this painting is almost too painful for comfort if you're a man past fifty. As the doctor explains where he's going to have to implant the replacement faucet, the patient squeezes his legs, curls his toes, pushes on himself, and eyes the doctor with a helpless look which only those who have ever been catheterized can understand.

What is going on in the painting on the wall? This is symbolic of a scene from the patient's life. His past sins are all there: drinking, carousing, and unsafe sex. A visit to the urologist—with its attendant "punishment"—must seem to the patient like a day in court.

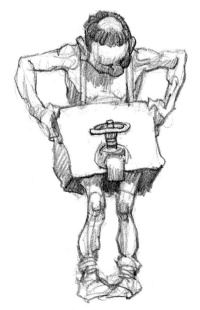

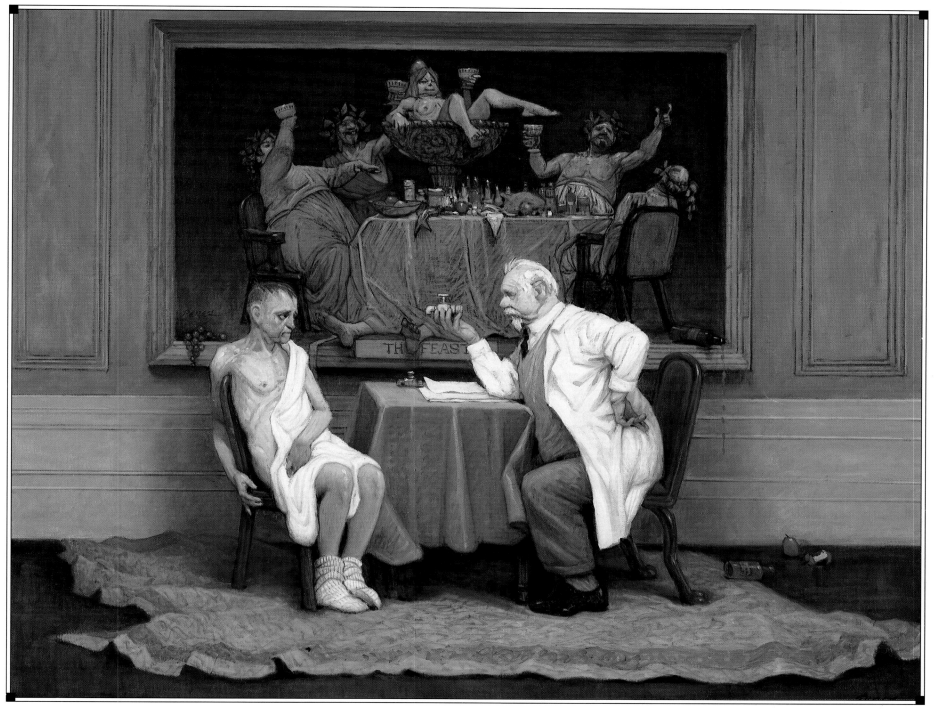

*T*he *U*rologist – 24" x 30" (61.5cm x 77cm)

THE VETERINARIAN

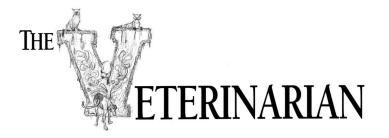

Perez has an unusual love for animals of all kinds, and it shows in this painting. His veterinarian has a kind and wise demeanor that would do justice to the veterinarian in **All Creatures Great and Small.**

With the baby orangutan clearly bawling out a high note as the doctor removes an offending splinter, the concerned creatures of the woods gather around to await the result with an empathy that perhaps only animals can show. Body language is certainly not limited to humans, and this work of art tells us that veterinary medicine has rewards that human medicine cannot share.

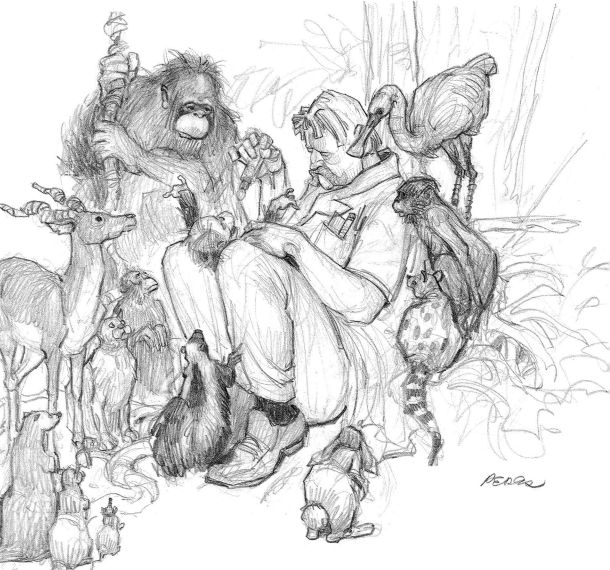

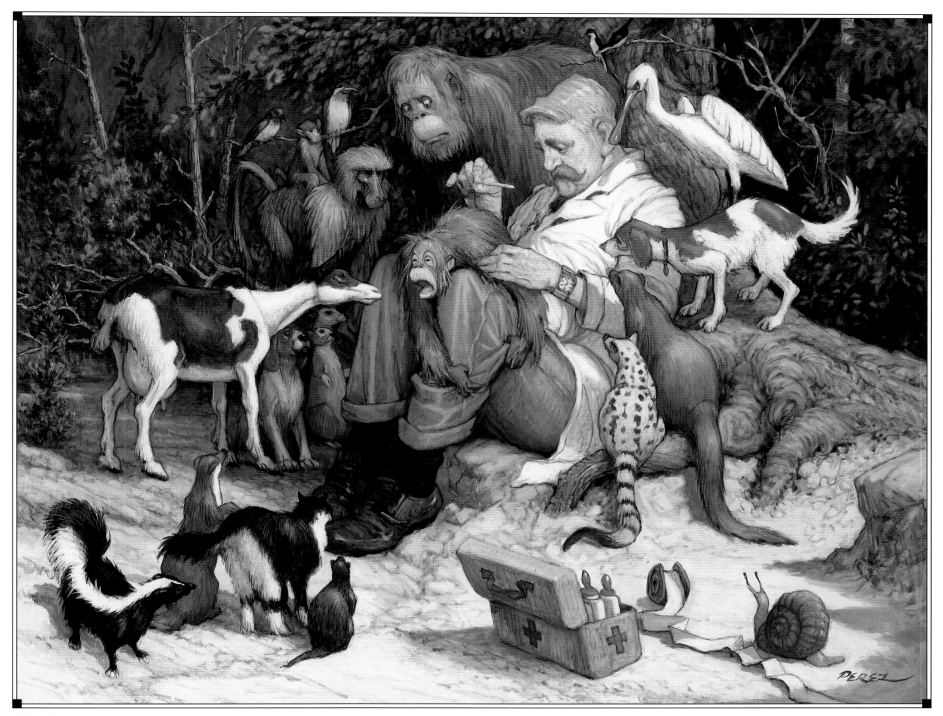

*T*he *V*eterinarian – 24" x 30" (61.5cm x 77cm)

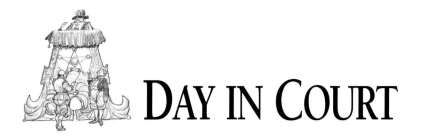

DAY IN COURT

This artistic commentary on the world of law is included in the series on medicine because the two professions are intrinsically linked together. Not only will one-third of all U.S. doctors be sued every year for malpractice, but defensive medicine results in billions of dollars of overtesting. Some fields of medicine, such as obstetrics, are losing frightened practitioners at an alarming rate. Poverty, child abuse, environmental neglect, discrimination, illiteracy, drug abuse, and other social ills all affect our health, and all involve both professions.

Perez painted "A Day in Court" after having spent a frustrating day in court himself over a minor legal dispute. The parables and metaphors of his insight are visible in every part of the canvas, and all sorts of engrossing subplots capture the attention of the viewer. Meanwhile, the whole scene comes together masterfully in the look on the face of the judge, who bears an unmistakable resemblance to Perez himself.

Persons viewing this painting seem to have different favorite characters, depending upon their own experiences. While Justice sleeps and the court jester does his tricks, practically every segment of society tries to get the attention of the judge for its own political needs. One can look at this painting for weeks and still discover fresh aspects which have remained previously unnoticed. Like characters in a parade, all the characters in this painting seem the same, and yet different.

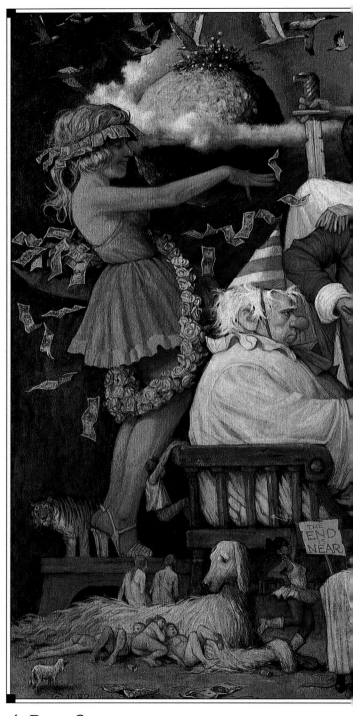

A Day in Court - 48" x 96" (123cm x 246cm)

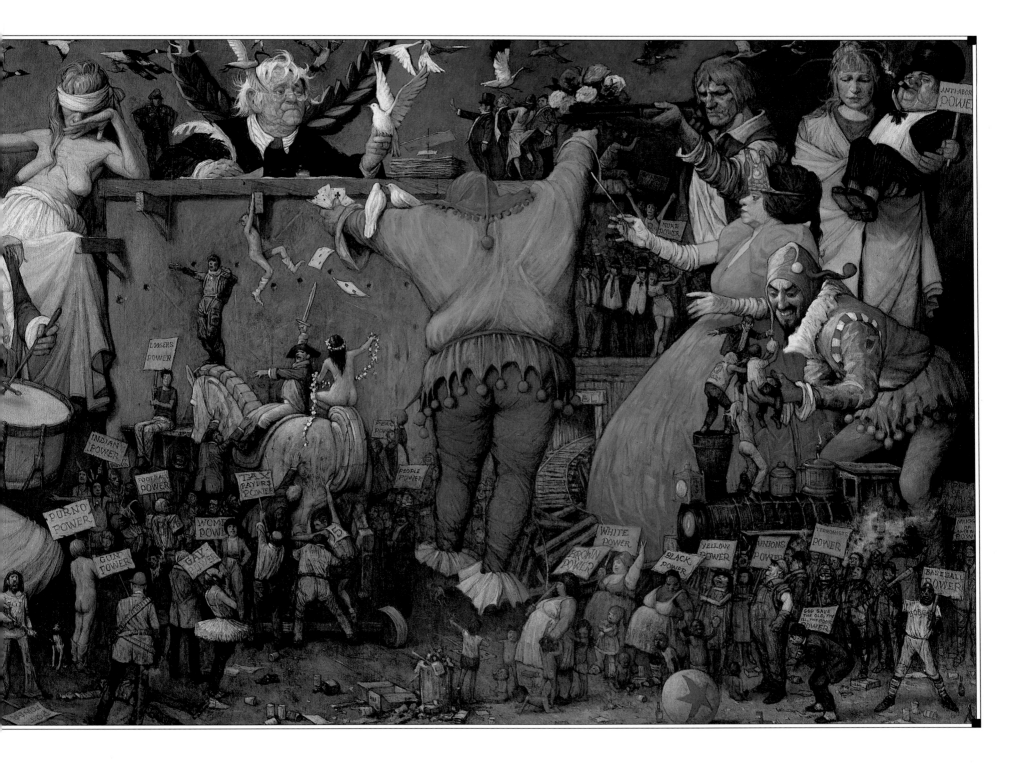

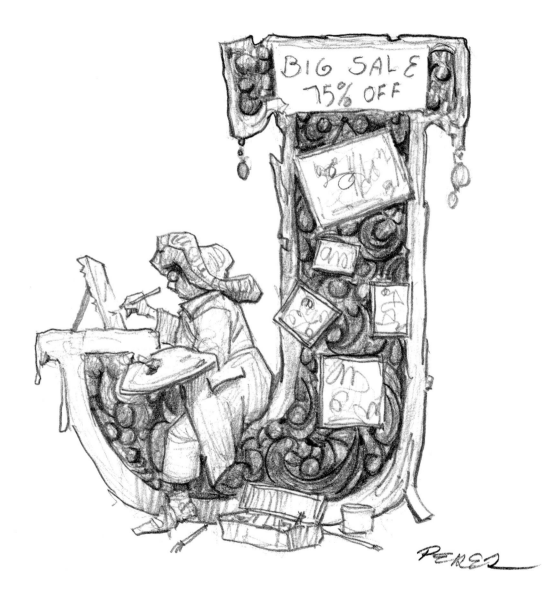